I0090966

Pregnancy Your Way

Pregnancy Your Way

Choose a Safe and Happy Birth

Dr. Alan R. Lindemann
with *Diane Haugen*

ARL, Inc.
P.O. Box 52 Elgin, ND 58533

Copyright ©2023 by ARL, Inc. First Edition 2023.

All Rights Reserved. No part of this book may be used, copied, or reproduced in any form without written permission except for the quoting of brief passages for review purposes.

Printed in the United States of America

Illustrations by Trygve Olson
Book design and production by www.AuthorSuccess.com

ISBN (paperback): 978-0-9632244-5-3
ISBN (ebook): 978-0-9632244-6-0

The information supplied in this book is not intended to be used as medical treatment or diagnosis. Dr. Alan R. Lindemann and ARL, Inc. make no representations or warranties regarding the content of this book and will not be held liable with respect to its accuracy, completeness, or usefulness.

DEDICATION

In residency, my attending physician listened to her patients more closely than many of the other physicians. Her attention to her patients became a model for the way I wanted to practice medicine and it has served me well.

My first clinical practice was in Crookston, MN, after finishing my residency in obstetrics and gynecology at Regions Hospital in Minneapolis, MN. I learned much from the nurses and doctors practicing there; solutions to real world problems that sometimes escape the medical school environment. Thankfully, the patients in Crookston were quick to trust a young doctor, and I listened to what they told me.

I dedicate this book to my many obstetric patients who have paved the way, enabling me to pass their insights on to the present generation of women contemplating or anticipating bringing a new life into the world.

Alan Lindemann, M.D.

Free offer to readers of this book:

There are a lot of birth plans available, but I believe your whole pregnancy deserves the same attention to detail that your birth plan deserves.

I have developed a series of questions you should be attending to from the very beginning when you are simply planning to become pregnant, continuing during your pregnancy, your labor and delivery, and most important of all, during the first year after you deliver. I call this attention to detail your *flight plan*.

This book continues to evolve as I add weekly blog posts to his LindemannMD.com web site at https://lindemannmd.com/blog/. If you would like to join the conversation, please check out PregnancyYourWay.com where you may register to ask questions and make comments.

Download a Free Sample Flight Plan!
https://dl.bookfunnel.com/oduchubfpk

CONTENTS

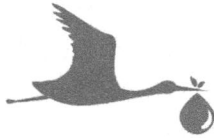

Protect Yourself and Your Baby

I knocked on the door and entered my exam room, where a twenty-five-year-old woman, eight weeks pregnant, had come for her first prenatal visit. My obstetric nurse had checked her vitals and taken her medical history.

"Good morning," I said as I entered the room. "I'm Dr. Lindemann. Thank you for stopping by."

"Good morning, Dr. Lindeman. I'm here to interview you." She'd been to two other obstetricians. "You are the third and final doctor, and after this visit I'll decide who I want to see for my prenatal and delivery care." She added "You've delivered three of my friends and they're happy with your care."

"Thank you for sharing that with me!" I said. "I'd like to begin by asking you if you have any questions for me."

Many first-time moms are often a little anxious, maybe even a little scared. I try to remove as much of the anxiety as possible from the interview. I sit in a chair away from my desk to be sure they can see me, and I want to see them. Body position is important during an interview. I don't cross my arms across my chest or stand in the doorway as if I'm trying to escape. I also don't want to see my patient cross her arms, either. Arm crossing signals the end of communication.

"Can my husband come along with me to my prenatal visits?" she asked.

Husbands on prenatal visits are one of my favorite topics. "Your husband is welcome. In fact, I prefer your husband to come to the visits with you. I like my patients and their husbands to experience pregnancy, delivery, and postpartum care together. It always helps when both of you have a better idea of what to expect all the way through to baby's first birthday and beyond."

"Will I see you every time I come in for an appointment and will you be present for my delivery?"

Another of my favorite topics. "Yes, I will see you for all your prenatal visits and for your delivery. I very seldom miss my patient deliveries.

My turn to ask questions: "How many brothers and sisters do you have?"

"I have one sister and two brothers," she replied.

Knowing how a patient's mother did in pregnancy is very helpful. "Did your mom have any difficulties with her deliveries?"

"My mother had no trouble with her pregnancies. She delivered us all at full term and without any anesthesia," she answered.

Then she asked, "What can you tell me about nausea and weight gain during pregnancy?"

"I've listened to many patients tell me how they ate to avoid nausea and vomiting during pregnancy. I've learned a lot from them. None of my patients has required supplemental feeding with a nose hose or IV nutrition." I went on to explain that I recommend my patients gain two or three pounds of weight each month. "At first, with nausea and possibly vomiting, it may be a bit of a challenge to gain weight, but by eight months, gaining two to three pounds a month might be too easy. You should eat about 120 to 130 grams of protein each day to prevent your body from using your muscle for protein."

"Most people today eat cold cereal, skim milk, a glass of juice, and toast for breakfast. This is a carbohydrate load. If that's all you eat, you'll be nauseated and most likely be vomiting in twenty or thirty minutes. If you are wedded to your cold cereal, I recommend adding whole milk, and having some full-fat yogurt, at least for the duration of your pregnancy. If you can handle eating a hard-boiled egg, that would be great. Hard boiled eggs provide the necessary protein and fat to balance the carbohydrates. You should have thirty to forty grams of protein with each big meal (three per day) and five to ten grams with your three or four smaller meals, for a total 120 to 130 grams per day.

"If you have a carbohydrate load, your sugar will go up and your pancreas will "kick in,' making a batch of insulin and abruptly dropping your sugar. That's when you will feel nauseated and will likely vomit.

"If you eat balanced meals, your blood sugar will remain more balanced, also. The goal of eating when you're pregnant is to keep your blood sugar under control, neither too high nor too low. The first half of your pregnancy is usually dominated by low blood sugar, with the second half of your pregnancy usually reflecting high blood sugar levels."

"This is more complicated than I thought!" she said. "I'm not sure I can remember all that."

"No problem," I responded. "I'll send you home with some written instructions. You can call anytime you need to, especially if you have trouble with nausea and vomiting."

She looked at me and smiled. Without hesitation, she

said, "We'll be returning to you for our prenatal care, Dr. Lindemann."

"Then today," I told her, "we'll draw some routine labs to measure your hemoglobin, kidney and liver function, thyroid levels, blood sugar, and antibodies. If all your labs are normal, my nurse Kathy will call you in one week. If there's anything abnormal in the labs, I will call you within the week and discuss the labs myself. When you come back in a month, we'll go over your labs and listen to your baby's heartbeat. Please bring your husband."

Before she left, I assured her that if she had any questions, she shouldn't hesitate to call my office. I was available to my patients twenty-four hours a day, seven days a week.

I'm now retired and have the opportunity to share what I have learned about safe pregnancies, deliveries, and postpartum with women and their families everywhere. I spend time now on social media; something I thought I would never do. But what I found surprised me. The postpartum troubles that young moms and dads are having, they shouldn't be having. To outsiders, these problems might seem to be small, like who should clean the breast pump, wash the dishes, get up with the baby, prepare meals, sleep in, clean the house, or go shopping.

But to the postpartum mom and dad, these problems are anything but small. They can turn your life upside down and inside out. What's more, the whole world says you should love this new little creature and even enjoy your duty caring for it. Until now, you, like many others, thought you could handle anything. But this is different. Just try being sleep deprived for a week or two. How's your emotional state? How do you feel about problem solving with sleep deprivation? To make matters worse, if you go without enough sleep for long enough, you might not even feel sleepy, just depressed or anxious, and sleeping might be difficult for many reasons.

Thirty years ago, these problems I now see posted on social media were less frequent. Why? We kept moms and babies in the hospital for three or more days, until we knew they were ready to go home. On morning rounds, we listened to our new moms and the nurses. Usually, we discussed whether a particular mom, baby, and husband or partner were ready to manage once home. Was your breastmilk in, could your baby latch on, was your baby gaining weight, were there any signs of jaundice, and of course, did mom and husband or significant other (SO) know what to expect when you got home? Had you and your husband or SO divided household chores at home? Who would be responsible for what? Today, with stays for vaginal deliveries shortened to twenty-four hours or less, sometimes your doctor has no way of knowing whether moms, babies, and dads or SOs are ready to go home.

I saw my patients every time they came to my clinic because I wanted to observe what strengths and problems they had and help them understand how taking responsibility for their own care would help bring about the outcomes they wanted in their pregnancy, delivery, and postpartum period. I believe my active participation in the care of my patients has always helped to improve my patients' outcomes.

Too many doctors don't take the time to listen to your story, your concerns, or thoroughly answer your questions. Too few doctors are willing to spend time working with nature but are too quick to induce labor or order a C-section. Both labor inductions and C-sections carry significant risks.

Your first job when you find out you are pregnant is to look for a doctor who will listen and answer your questions. Many of my patients came to me because I would listen to what they had to say when others would not. To tell the truth, my advice on how to manage nausea in pregnancy is based largely upon what I learned by listening to my patients. This is information that isn't in medical textbooks and may not be the information you can get from your obstetrician. The information I provide here is meant to be shared with your doctor, not be a replacement for medical advice.

A lot of your questions about pregnancy don't necessarily fit neatly into a timeline. You may have questions about blood pressure during your first or third trimester. So, I have arranged this book a bit differently than many books on pregnancy. The major subjects in your pregnancy can be found in the Table of Contents. You won't find information here about whether you should be drinking coffee while you're pregnant or how you can keep stretch marks to a minimum (bad news—they're a given) because there are many very good "encyclopedias" of data about every aspect of pregnancy. You'll find some of these references listed at the end of this book.

The "one-size-fits-all" notion of pregnancy and delivery may leave you with a lot of questions about your pregnancy. Any book will emphasize the importance of keeping your blood pressure in a normal range during your pregnancy. However, something as simple as blood pressure varies significantly from one pregnancy to another, something your physician should share with you. In Chapter 2, you will find out what you need to know about blood pressure during your pregnancy. In fact, you will learn that you really need to know what your blood pressure is before you get pregnant because you need a benchmark for monitoring your blood pressure during pregnancy.

Each chapter provides you with space to record helpful information and a place to record questions you may want to ask on your next prenatal visit. At the end our book you will find lists of online resources about your pregnancy, a list of organizations which support women in pregnancy, and a list of references.

My goal in writing this book is to provide you with the information you need to feel confident about your pregnancy and feel assured in your ability to ask questions you need to make the decisions best for you:

- how to find the right doctor for you,

- how to make decisions with your doctor

- how to advocate for yourself in the healthcare system
- how to take care of yourself, and
- how to create a birth plan, or as I like to think of it, a flight plan

Here, I provide information you need to have confidence in yourself and never be afraid to ask questions, no matter how small they may seem to you. You will find the information you need to make your flight plan and work with your physician to put together a plan which will work best for you.

You may download my suggestions for what information should be included in your birth plan. I like to call this information a *flight plan* because it covers prenatal care through labor and delivery, not just your few hours in the hospital to deliver your baby. In fact, I like your flight plan to include something missing in most plans for your baby—information to help you through the first year after our baby is born.

Think Air Force One with your flight plan. Your flight plan with your baby as passenger is every bit as important as the passenger of Air Force One, the President of the United States.

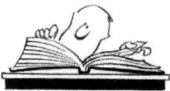

REFERENCES

"How to Create a Birth Plan - Planning for Labor and Delivery," WebMD, accessed May 2, 2023, https://www.webmd.com/baby/guide/how-to-create-a-birth-plan.

Liz Says, et al., "Writing a Birth Plan: 10 Essential Tips from a Pediatrician and Mom of 5," ChildrensMD, August 19, 2013, https://childrensmd.org/uncategorized/writing-a-birth-plan-10-essential-tips-from-a-pediatrician-and-mom-of-5/.

SECTION 1

You're in Charge of Your Pregnancy

Sarah, my receptionist, rang: "Dr. Lindemann, you have a new patient with four babies in her uterus (quads). Her name is Sandy. When would you like to see her? I think she's been doctor shopping."

"Put her on the schedule today at noon so I can spend all the time I need to with her."

Sandy and Doug arrived shortly before noon, and I went to the waiting room to greet them and take them to my office.

"How did you find me?" I asked Sandy.

"We went to Mothers of Multiples and asked which doctor had the most experience with multiples, and your name came up most often."

I could see that Sandy and Doug were anxious. I did not send the wrong body language signals to them that might worry them more than they were already.

Sandy and Doug were well dressed and articulate. Sandy said, "You are our fourth doctor interview. We have quads as a result of in vitro fertilization. We've been to three doctors in two cities who have recommended that we decrease the number of babies from four to two."

"They call that *reduction*," Doug said, "but we can't make that choice."

I wanted to be sure they understood what was going on in this situation. I asked, "Do you know why you are getting the reduction recommendation?"

"I think there are two reasons," Sandy said. "First, they think I will have a better chance of carrying twins longer than quads, and second, quads are a mistake from their viewpoint."

"I think that both of you understand well the reasons that these three doctors have recommended **reduction**," I said. "But you are still in this moral dilemma, which nobody has addressed. You can't act on these recommendations. They are irrelevant for you.

"Please correct me if I misunderstand, but you're telling me that your pregnancy is going to be all or nothing. Are you prepared for those two possible outcomes?"

Doug replied, "Yes, all four get the same chance to live or not to live, but they will all be treated equally."

This decision would last a lifetime.

Doug, Sandy and I discussed planning for this pregnancy, including labs, ultrasounds, prenatal visits, and smoking less with maximum benefit for the quads.

Sandy smoked cigarettes. I said, "You need to quit!"

She said, "I can't!"

"Let's compromise," I said. "Sometimes nobody gets exactly what they want. But let's try a win-win. If you smoke one cigarette a day, I win because that's less than you now smoke, and you win because one is better than none. Smoking less is the first of many compromises I'll ask for from now on.

"Today, if you decide to stay with me, before you leave, I want to do an ultrasound to make sure that there are four babies and four beating hearts. I will see you weekly so that we can adjust your birth plan, or what I call your 'flight plan,' as needed."

Sandy's pregnancy went along well for the first twenty-eight weeks. She called at about twenty-eight weeks and said, "I can't eat."

I hospitalized her for a day to give her some nutrition, some hydration, and to try to discover what was happening to her, and to see if things could be turned around for her.

Sandy stayed in the hospital for one day and then I sent her home to see if she might be able to resume eating. The next morning, I got another call from Sandy, "I still can't eat."

I put Sandy back in the hospital again after I saw her in my office and did another pelvic exam. She spent the night in the hospital again and I went to see her the next morning.

"How are you doing Sandy?" I asked.

"I still can't eat, and I don't feel very good," she replied.

The nurses were in the room with us. I checked Sandy's cervix. It was completely closed but had thinned (effaced) about 50 percent of what was needed for labor. I saw no contractions.

The day went by, and I got no calls from the nurses about Sandy. I called the hospital several times and was told that nothing was happening. About midnight, a nurse called and said, "Sandy has back pain."

"Check her cervix," I told the nurse. In a panic, the nurse returned my call five minutes later saying, "Sandy's complete!"

That meant her cervix was dilated about ten centimeters and she was ready to deliver all four babies.

In fifteen minutes, I raced across town in the January snow and ice of North Dakota.

After fifteen or twenty minutes, we were in the operating room with its bright lights, anesthesiologists, Sandy, Doug, and four neonatologists. At least fifteen people were in that room.

Sandy was given a spinal for anesthesia.

Finally came my part. With so many babies so small, they needed to be delivered by C-section. They all weighed about a pound and a half; normal for their gestational age. The four babies were sent to the neonatal intensive care unit and did well.

Sandy has kept me informed over the years. The quads grew up well. I saw their graduation and holiday family pictures. It was indeed a pleasure to see them all healthy and well. This result goes back to the first day with the moral decision that Sandy and Doug made at their first visit. The quads would be treated equally. Sandy and Doug decided it was all or nothing, but whatever happened, the result was going to be fair.

I've heard people say that obstetrics is 98 percent boredom and 2 percent terror. I disagree. Years of delivering healthy babies from healthy moms has shown me obstetrics should be 100 percent looking for subtle signs of developing problems and addressing the problems before they become disasters.

Birth plans, a common fixture in the reading material for pregnant women, cover discussing your wants and needs for delivery with your obstetrician. While the process of creating a birth plan with your obstetrician is very valuable, this plan only covers a few days of your pregnancy. What women really need is a *flight plan;* a birth plan for your entire pregnancy and the twelve months after you deliver your baby. Think about it. You, the mother, are the pilot and your obstetrician the copilot. As the pilot of your pregnancy, you must keep an eye on all kinds of gauges or measurements that you, as the pilot, with the help of your baby's dad and your obstetrician, need to monitor for a safe pregnancy. At the same time, you have a passenger, your baby, back in the passenger section. A birth plan certainly covers the delivery of your passenger in your flight plan's landing. But you need a flight plan for your entire pregnancy and for a year after you deliver your baby, not just a birth plan.

To me, closely monitoring a pregnancy in cooperation with the expectant mother and father feels much like steering a pregnancy. Women need to feel comfortable with taking part in this steering process along with their copilot, the obstetrician.

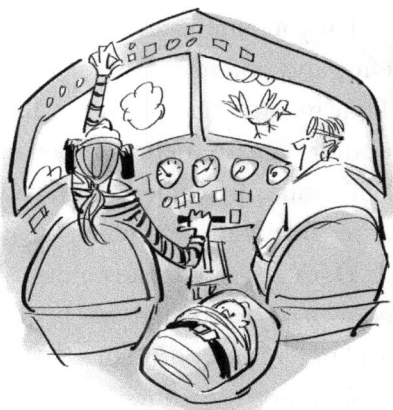

Understand the Role of Informed Consent

Most people have heard of informed consent. Who hasn't appeared for a clinic appointment and had sheets of paper shoved at you during check in? Does anyone really read those sheets before signing them? And if you do read them, what would happen if you found a clause you didn't like and asked for it to be removed? Would any healthcare organization allow you to selectively draw lines through some clauses and initial the deletions? Doubtful, which leads you to just sign whatever they're given.

Informed consent is not about giving health care organizations free reign in what they do to you. It's about choice—your choice.

Hospitals and payers (including insurance companies, Health Maintenance Organizations, Preferred Provider Organizations, Medicare, and Medicaid) have greatly eroded your choice and, indeed, your physician's choice. These healthcare conglomerates have usurped your ability to have the final say on whether treatment will be covered or not, and to choose which physicians you see.

For you, informed consent means understanding the purpose, benefits, and potential risks of the care being offered by your physician. That means your physician helps you to understand the treatment options you are being offered and the risks with the various options. With your physician's input, you should be able to choose a mutually agreeable treatment plan.

Does this sound like fantasy? Well, for many of us it is, because the control of health care has been taken out of the hands of physicians and put in the control of payers who make decisions based on saving money, not your physician's ability to provide the health care that's best for you.

A key element of informed consent is your ability to have the final say in what care you choose, even if the physician believes another choice would be better. Physicians are required to support your decisions.

When thinking of informed consent, most people don't think of choice as part of the equation. The next time you are at the doctor's office and asked to sign paperwork, think choice—then make yours.

Beware of "Evidence-Based" Medicine

Many statements about medical care today are prefaced with the new popular notion of "evidence-based" medicine. There's the implication that medical care is somehow flawed if there isn't some research paper somewhere indicating that the care offered is based upon some research study. Patient care is becoming more and more like a cookbook recipe. If the physician checks off everything on the recipe as okay, the assumption is that there's nothing wrong. It seems that medical schools no longer teach physicians to continue the search for a diagnosis even if the recipe turns up no problems. As I've said before, the notion of "one size fits all" does not fit pregnancy. Nowhere is this a more important concept than in obstetrics. Obstetrics isn't about disease. It's about preserving the good health of you and your baby; about choosing your outcome and achieving what you want.

I considered a couple of specialties when I was in medical school, but I soon realized in my obstetrical rotation one thing that made obstetrics different from other specialties. In obstetrics, it wasn't just a matter of identifying and curing a disease. The doctor and the parents could aim for a desired outcome, a healthy baby. Yes, mothers and fathers can choose to have a healthy baby. That's steering the pregnancy. All doctors want to have successful treatments and surgeries, but obstetrics has more impact on future life. There are two patients, not one. A healthy baby's birth has consequences for the lives of many people for years to come.

Though physical and emotional health challenges may present during pregnancy and soon after birth—from eclampsia to postpartum depression—it is possible to decrease the effects of these potentially dangerous conditions with the help of an attentive physician. You can choose the goal of being a healthy mother and having a healthy baby and then act to steer the pregnancy in that direction. It may seem that maternal health is left up to biology and chance, but the truth is that many of the challenges pregnant women face can be managed or even prevented.

Knowing that we can choose our goals as we put together your pregnancy flight plan makes it possible to keep what we want and to change much of what we don't want. For example, nausea and anorexia become manageable. Management means eating the right things at the right time for the right weight gain. Knowing that blood pressure is manageable can add safety and duration to your pregnancy. In other words, the pregnancy can get closer to term, adding safety for your baby. Under no circumstances should babies be sent home when there is nothing for them to eat. Then there is depression, which can be managed with medications and practical lifestyle adjustments. Let's not have postpartum depression or psychosis.

Hospital CEOs and payers pressure physicians to send new mothers home before their milk comes in. This is an insurance ploy to "save money." On the books, it may look like this saves the hospital lots of money, but many of these babies wind up readmitted to the hospital for "failure to thrive," a term which might as well be called starvation. Moms and dads need to know when to supplement breast milk with formula, although lactation specialists often prefer there be no formula given. There is also the option of expressing breast milk with a pump and allowing dads to feed their babies.

Designing a flight plan for the whole pregnancy and the months after the delivery of the baby helps moms, dads, and babies do better. In many cases we can avoid prematurity, strokes, seizures, eclampsia, liver and kidney damage, and death. Of the 850 maternal deaths per year in the United States, experts agree that 45 percent of those deaths are preventable. Obstetricians should be trained to understand what it is to steer a pregnancy to avoid some of these preventable maternal deaths. You may need to see your doctor more often than the allotted visits per pregnancy paid for by your insurance company. Ask your physician on your initial interview how any extra visits are handled.

Flight Plan Considerations

A good place to start your flight plan is with choosing obstetricians to visit and putting together the questions you would like to ask during your interviews. For suggestions about the kinds of things to consider in a flight plan, download my free Flight Plan.

There will be surprises in your pregnancy, but thankfully, many of the surprises can be managed well by you, the pilot of your flight plan. Use the information in this book to help you build your and your baby's flight plan, covering your plans for your prenatal care, your labor and delivery, and your first year after your baby is born.

You Can Manage Your Body's Response to Your Pregnancy

Ever wonder the kinds of things obstetricians monitor during your pregnancy? Or at least are supposed to monitor? With the corporate takeover of medicine by people with no medical background, many of the ways obstetricians once tracked patient progress have disappeared. If you have a problem or a concern, chances are you won't be scheduled to see your obstetrician, but rather you will talk to a nurse practitioner or a nurse. What's more, you have no way of knowing if your concerns are passed on to your obstetrician. Part of what you should have looked for in your choice of obstetricians is one who will be available to answer your questions personally, even if it's over the phone. Or by means of telemedicine. The pandemic has at least made it possible for patients to visit their physicians online. Your search for a physician should include finding an obstetrical practice where your questions don't fall between the cracks. This section covers the major signs and signals obstetricians should be monitoring in your pregnancy. There's nothing to prevent you from monitoring these indicators, as well. In fact, the information you gather may well fill in some important gaps which might otherwise be missed in the standard office visits during your pregnancy. The topics covered in this chapter include:

- blood pressure,

- preeclampsia,

- morning sickness,

- exercise,

- headaches,

- nonstress tests,

- hormones, and

- stress and anxiety.

It's important for you to monitor those pregnancy markers you can at home so that you can let your physician know about a possible problem right away instead of waiting for the next scheduled visit. Blood pressure, the first factor on the list, is a very important marker of how well your pregnancy is progressing. As noted in the Introduction, the chapters in this book are designed to be read in any order depending upon what topic may be on your mind.

With one exception—the chapter on blood pressure!

In my experience in 6,000 deliveries, I have come to believe that my close attention to blood pressure fluctuations in my patients had a lot to do with my success in avoiding maternal mortalities.

CHAPTER 1

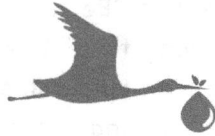

Blood Pressure

I met Alicia for the first time when she had come into labor and delivery (the area of the hospital designated for deliveries) at term. She had been followed by one of the approximately thirty family practice doctors I worked with. Her doctor had called me and asked me to see Alicia. Her blood pressure was 130/90. From her records I could see that her initial pressure was 90/50. Her lab indicated worsening kidney and liver functions, with low platelets. When I went to see her, I asked, "How do you feel?"

"I don't feel bad," she said. "I don't have any pain anywhere."

"I want to listen to your lungs and to check your reflexes. Is that okay?" I asked. "The nurse said your cervix is closed, so I don't need to recheck that. Your baby appears to be in good shape according to your monitor."

Alicia's lungs were clear. No evidence of pulmonary edema or congestive heart failure. Her reflexes were very active with some clonus, which means after tapping her knee, instead of one kick, there were several. I reported to Alicia, "You have a significant elevation of blood pressure and very active reflexes, meaning that you have preeclampsia. I want to deliver you soon. Your baby is ready. I don't want you to have a seizure or a stroke."

I knew I needed to explain to her why I was recommending a cesarean section. "Because your cervix is closed induction could take a long time," I said. "You could have a seizure or a stroke from an epidural, so I want to go ahead and do a C-section. Do you understand?"

Alicia answered, "I think so, but I don't feel bad. I didn't know I was so sick."

I didn't tell Alicia at that time how worried I was about her physical condition. In residency we learn not to frighten our patients, something most of us do. Anxiety can seriously interfere with labor. Patients need to feel they are the only person who matters at the time.

"We'll be doing general anesthesia, which means you'll be going to sleep for your C-section," I said. "With your blood pressure higher than it should be and your lab values indicating you have severe preeclampsia, we need to deliver your baby without a long induction."

I wasn't worried about the general anesthesia because I had a good anesthetist, and I knew I could get the baby out in two minutes or less.

In approximately half an hour Alicia, was on the operating table ready for surgery. Vitals including the fetal heart rate, were stable. Within another thirty seconds the breathing tube was in place and I could start the surgery. The baby was born approximately two minutes later with Apgars of 8+ 9+ and weighed 7 lbs. 10 oz. Alicia's vitals remained stable during the surgery and her blood loss was minimal. The surgical closure repair took approximately fifteen minutes.

Alicia awakened easily. Blood loss remained minimal. Her pressure remained constant. To treat her hypertension and pre-eclampsia post-operatively, I began IV apresoline, propranolol, and magnesium sulfate. Alicia did well post-operatively. Each day her pressure came down a bit, as expected.

On the fifth day, I sent her home on oral apresoline and propranolol. Three days later, Alicia came to my office for a scheduled post-partum visit. Her blood pressure was 110/75, her incision was doing well, and her baby was eating and gaining weight. Kidney and liver function had returned to normal. She returned for another scheduled post-operative visit a week later. She was still doing well and scheduled a follow-up visit with her family practice doctor after that.

Alicia was a very sick young lady who could have had many problems, but with careful attention, she did not have a stroke, liver damage, kidney damage, paralysis, or nursing home placement.

Serious illness starting out as rising blood pressure should not end tragically. In my experience, addressing increasing blood pressure in pregnancy is 100 percent treatable.

It's important for you to monitor those pregnancy markers you can at home so you can let your physician know about a possible problem right away instead of waiting for the next scheduled visit. Blood pressure, the first factor on the list, is a very important marker of how well your pregnancy is progressing. As noted in the Introduction, the chapters in this book are designed to be read in any order depending upon what topic may be on your mind.

With one exception—this chapter on blood pressure!

In my experience with 6,000 deliveries, I have come to believe that my close attention to blood pressure fluctuations in my patients had a lot to do with my success in avoiding maternal mortalities.

If you read nothing else in this book, read the information presented here on hypertension in pregnancy. Many of the stories on the internet about pregnancies and deliveries gone wrong start with blood pressure which was overlooked, ignored, or misunderstood.

Managing your blood pressure is the best way to achieve a healthy baby. This chapter will explain one way you can avoid becoming a story on the internet: Track your blood pressure yourself at home from the very beginning of your pregnancy. In fact, establish what your normal blood pressure is **BEFORE** you become pregnant. Managing your blood pressure is one of the best ways to have a healthy baby.

It's the High Blood Pressure That Counts!

Years ago, I sent my patients with elevated blood pressure to labor and delivery. The nurses would place the patient in the left lateral decubitus position (midway between back and left side) and over a period of time, take their blood pressure fifteen times. They would then call me and report the lowest blood pressure, tell me all was normal, and send the patient home. The patients would return to my clinic a week later with even higher blood pressures, making their pregnancies harder to manage.

Early in my obstetric life, I learned that the lowest blood pressure seldom meant anything. Rather, the highest blood pressure has the most predictive value. Treating that highest blood pressure value early was often simple. I had my patients check their own blood pressure daily at home. All that was required was the purchase of a $50 blood pressure cuff.

Blood pressure monitoring needs to be taken in the context of your first blood pressure reading. Blood pressure will almost always be lower at around week twelve or twenty of your pregnancy. So, your blood pressure at twelve to twenty weeks is going to be as good as it gets. Blood pressures usually stay low until about thirty weeks, at which time they will return to pre-pregnancy values. Sometimes blood pressure will start to go up at twenty weeks.

What to Watch for With Your Blood Pressure

A patient presented at my office for her first pregnancy visit. Her blood pressure was 150/90. I asked myself what I would do with a blood pressure like this so early in pregnancy.

I had two problems. I had to consider how I might treat this patient with this kind of blood pressure if she weren't pregnant, and also consider how I could treat this kind of blood pressure when she was pregnant. Fortunately, her blood pressure dropped in the first trimester of her pregnancy. I prescribed Aldomet. Her pressure remained 130/80 throughout her pregnancy. She delivered a 9 lb. 2 oz. boy at term. No preeclampsia.

How to Manage Your Blood Pressure at Home

My experience helping women manage blood pressures at home dates back to 1980. As I've said so often, there is no one-size-fits all, and that is particularly true of blood pressures in pregnancy. Blood pressure can vary from high to low. **CONTEXT IS EVERYTHING**.

Each patient is different. Depending upon their blood pressures, I had some patients come to the office for checks twice a week, some of them every other day, or in some cases, every day. How frequently I had my patients come to the office for blood pressure checks depended most often upon three criteria:

- the patient's blood pressure was high at the start of pregnancy,

- the patient's blood pressure was high during the office visit, and

- how far along the patient was in her pregnancy.

High Blood Pressure Before Pregnancy

Please be sure to know your blood pressure before you become pregnant. It would be a good idea to ask your doctor how he or she treats slowly rising blood pressure during pregnancy. If you are told your doctor waits until your upper blood pressure number is 160 before treating you, you might consider interviewing some more doctors before choosing which one you choose to oversee your pregnancy.

Some women will start a pregnancy with blood pressure in the normal range, only to have it increase as the pregnancy progresses. In my experience, there are four kinds of hypertension related to pregnancy:

- hypertension prior to pregnancy, controlled during pregnancy,
- hypertension new to pregnancy without pre-eclampsia,
- hypertension new to pregnancy with pre-eclampsia, and
- hypertension before pregnancy and made worse by pregnancy.

There's been a lot of criticism from some healthcare workers that home blood pressure cuffs just cause people to go to the ER unnecessarily. Just the same, if you begin to see signs of your blood pressure going up, you can talk with your doctor about what that means for you in your pregnancy. Blood pressure is relative and, in my experience, begins rising slowly in pregnancy. If your systolic blood pressure (the top number) goes up more than ten points, it's time to talk with your doctor about the appearance of hypertension in your pregnancy.

CHAPTER 2

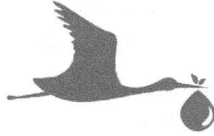

Preeclampsia

Preeclampsia, strictly speaking, is diagnosed when there is a combination of elevated blood pressure, protein in your urine (indicating kidney failure), hyperreflexia (knee extends more than once with tapping), and lab signs of other organ failure. But in my experience, there are other factors involved, as well:

- serum creatinine,

- urine leukocytes (white cells) and protein,

- hemoglobin/hematocrit (Hgb/HCT),

- liver function tests (LFTs), alanine aminotransferase (ALT), aspartate aminotransferase (AST), alkaline phosphatase (ALP), and

- platelets.

Preeclampsia is an illness strictly related to pregnancy. It is a multi-system disorder that affects 2 to 5 percent of pregnant women. It is one of the leading causes of maternal and infant mortality worldwide. Each year, 76,000 mothers and 500,000 babies die from the effects of preeclampsia.

We don't really know why some women develop preeclampsia and some do not. However, the current theory suggests a two-phase process having to do with the way the placenta implants into the uterus. In early pregnancy, the placenta does not attach deeply enough to the uterus. At about seven to eight weeks, as the placenta grows and develops, preeclampsia might develop in response to the placenta's inability to lodge deeply enough into the uterus.

If these lab values are out of normal range for pregnancy and left unaddressed, a patient will possibly develop HELLP syndrome, which consists of the following symptoms:

- hemolysis, rupturing of red blood cells (H),
- elevated liver enzymes, indicating liver is not working properly (EL), and
- low platelets (LP).

There are several risks for your developing preeclampsia during your pregnancy:

- a family history of preeclampsia,
- preeclampsia in a previous pregnancy,
- chronic high blood pressure,
- high blood sugar,
- kidney disease, and
- autoimmune diseases such as lupus.

I once had a patient with HELLP (Hemolysis, Elevated Liver enzymes and Low Platelets) syndrome. She had mildly elevated blood pressure (130/85). I was watching her closely, checking blood creatinine, blood urea nitrogen, liver function, and urine protein.

She was, however, three days short of forty weeks gestation and had a favorable cervix. This was fortunate because the only treatment available for HELLP is delivery of the baby. We induced labor with Pitocin, the delivery went well, and I watched her in the hospital for four days after delivery. Her blood pressure and lab values returned to normal, and I sent her home with instructions to check her blood pressure two times each day and to come to the office to be checked in three days and seven days for follow up. Mom, dad, and baby did well, and as far as I know lived happily ever after.

The news recently carried a report of a young woman of color, a third- year pediatric resident, who died four days post-partum.[1] The article was short and had no real information except that she died on the fourth day postpartum from liver capsule rupture. The resident's excuse was that the patient had an unremarkable course, so they were surprised to find her suddenly dead.

The Symptoms of Preeclampsia

The primary problem with preeclampsia is that there are no signs or symptoms of early or moderately advanced illness. For severe preeclampsia, symptoms include headaches, visual disturbances, and right upper quadrant (liver) pain.

Contrary to what some people say or think, in my experience, preeclampsia does not come on suddenly. Onset might seem sudden, but only if we ignore subtle symptoms. Finding subtle signs early prevents patients with preeclampsia from progressing to eclampsia (seizures), hypertension, strokes, liver and kidney failure, paralysis, or death.

Diagnosing Preeclampsia

In my experience, the first and most subtle sign of preeclampsia is slightly elevated blood pressure. For example, if your BP is 110/70 (normal) during your middle trimester (fourteen to twenty-eight weeks), but increases to 116/75, that's a very subtle sign that your BP may be increasing. If you aren't already checking your blood pressure daily, you need to get a blood pressure cuff for home and check your pressure twice a day, once at eight in the morning and once at eight in the evening, and more often if you think you need to. Call your doctor (or phone nurse) if your pressure goes up ten points either diastolic (bottom number) or systolic (top number).

If you find your pressure is going up preterm, that's the time to adjust your schedule; for example, if you work three twelve hour shifts you should probably change to five seven-hour days. Working fewer hours per day is very beneficial for controlling blood pressure and managing preeclampsia.

How Preeclampsia Worsens

Years ago, we thought there was mild, moderate, and severe preeclampsia. Now it's more like mild or severe.[2] When dealing with preeclampsia, it is much better to think of it as a matter of degree, like shades of gray, not black or white. Finding preeclampsia early and treating it easily is our best option. In pregnancy, bed rest should be avoided, but with preeclampsia, you can still cut back on your work hours and increase your rest periods.

Your preeclampsia will worsen if your blood pressure is not controlled. As preeclampsia worsens, your blood pressure and lab results will continue to show increasingly harmful results. If your doctor tells you that you have preeclampsia and it is getting worse, your doctor should order the usual blood tests, which include a complete blood count, hemoglobin, and platelets, plus a comprehensive metabolic profile to look for kidney and liver functions, urinalysis for the presence of protein, and a D dimer (a test for abnormal blood coagulation). Except for the urine test, the other ones are blood draws. Your doctor should also order an ultrasound to see how big your baby is and to look at your amniotic fluid levels. If the fluid is low, that's another potential problem.

During Pregnancy, Lab Values Differ from "Normal"

I want to spend some time talking about hypertension *preceding* pregnancy, which can either improve or get worse during your pregnancy. Placing blood pressure in context is complicated, because what constitutes normal lab values when you are not pregnant do not constitute normal lab values when you are pregnant. Common labs such as blood urea nitrogen (BUN), hemoglobin (Hgb), and white blood count (WBC) are different depending upon whether you are pregnant or not.

TEST

NON-PREGNANT NORMAL
Hgb	12-16
Creatinine	0.7, 0.8, 0.9, 1.0

PREGNANT NORMAL
Hgb	11-12
Creatinine	0.5, 0.6, 0.7, 0.9

Using normal lab readings for pregnant women, without consideration for what the lab readings should be during pregnancy, might lead to poor outcomes for you.

Treatments for Preeclampsia

The best and most effective treatment for preeclampsia is early management of blood pressure. If your blood pressure starts to go up, your doctor may give you Aldomet, a blood pressure medication safe for you to take while you're pregnant.

The treatment for preeclampsia is delivery of your baby.

With even mild blood pressure elevations, I would recommend at least weekly visits for you. If your blood pressure isn't controlled and the other symptoms of preeclampsia progress, delivery or your baby is the only treatment. Once your pregnancy has reached at least thirty-two weeks, your baby has a good chance of survival.

If your hemoglobin is high, liver function and kidney functions have deteriorated, you need to get delivered. If your cervix is favorable and your baby is headfirst, vaginal birth by induction is the best option. In labor, you may get magnesium sulfate to mitigate preeclampsia and help prevent seizures. In my experience, magnesium sulfate acts as a tocolytic (stops labor), so you've got to deal with that problem. Other medications that you might be given to control your blood pressure in or after labor include apresoline and propranolol.

Unfortunately, all these medications can cross the placenta and effect your baby. Since propranolol is designed to decrease (control) mother's heart rate, it will also decrease your baby's heart rate postpartum. I have given as little medication as possible to a mother in labor so that the baby is not adversely affected by the medication. Once the baby is delivered, the mother's blood pressure can be decreased to about 130/80 to prevent stroke and death. But we certainly do not want blood pressure to be 110/70. Lowering blood pressure too fast decreases blood supply to vital organs.

Coping with a Preeclampsia Diagnosis

The best time to manage preeclampsia is before it gets to be a problem. If you have preeclampsia, work with your doctor to manage your blood pressure, watch your activity, and see your doctor regularly (at least once a week, if not more often).

Early observation and modified activity can protect you, as it has for my patients hundreds of times. Preeclampsia is most often reversible, treatable, and usually harmless IF MANAGED in time. It's the complications that make it difficult to treat, such as extreme hypertension (which causes strokes, paralysis, death), HELLP syndrome, liver capsule rupture, kidney failure, or liver failure.

If you develop preeclampsia, you'll need help managing the activities of daily living such as cleaning bathrooms, vacuuming floors, doing dishes, and making meals. Both you and your husband or SO need to plan for a division of labor before delivery and before you go home after delivery. After you are home from the hospital, you do not want to fight about who washes the breast pump or who gets up with the baby at night.

Many first-time mothers have mothers who can be helpful. If you have somebody coming into your house to help out, their job is to take care of the house. Someone needs to do the housework while you take care of your baby.

Much postpartum advice is practical. Postpartum adjustment today is more trouble than it used to be, partly because years ago mothers and dads had enough time to prepare for going home from the hospital after delivery. Sometimes mothers aren't ready to be mothers and dads aren't ready to be dads. There is a steep learning curve for first time mothers and dads after the delivery of the baby. Both before and after delivery you're going to need to rely on your husband or SO, or family members. If you cannot rely on help, then you might need counseling to avoid postpartum depression.

Preeclampsia Risk Highest After Delivery

It's often assumed that once the baby is delivered, the possibility of eclampsia subsides. But it doesn't always work that way. The postpartum time can be the worst time for blood pressure elevations. Your blood pressure should be monitored for fourteen days after delivery, or as long as it takes for your blood pressure to return to normal. It's possible a new mother may need to take anti-hypertensives for weeks, months, or even for the rest of her life.

I have had no patients with eclampsia (seizures due to preeclampsia) in my practice. I learned that vigilance must extend beyond the time of delivery. Blood pressure is individualized. Having a blood pressure of 150/100 is too high. Even after delivery you will need to keep in touch with your obstetrician or midwife if your blood pressure goes up more than ten points, either systolic (top number) or diastolic (bottom number) from your baseline.

The worst preeclampsia, eclampsia, and HELLP occur after delivery. That reality was firmly implanted in my mind. When a young mother dies four days post-partum, it is most likely due to either a saddle embolus, which is hard to detect, or liver rupture associated with HELLP. A saddle embolus shuts off all blood to the lungs. The outcome for a saddle embolus is universally bad. Despite immediate support to oxygenate blood or remove the lung clot, patients do not survive. Even if the clot is removed, they bleed to death. The best way to deal with the possibility of a saddle embolus is to look for clotting disorders or birth difficulties, personal or familial, before delivery. If clotting risks are established, you should be tested for D-Dimer and treated with Lovenox.

HELLP
(hemolysis, elevated liver enzymes,
low platelet count)

The ruptured liver capsule is more predictable and avoidable. The signs of HELLP are hemolysis (rupturing of blood vessels), elevated liver enzymes, and low platelets. With preeclampsia, you need to work with your doctor to address the problem before your preeclampsia evolves into the liver rupture of HELLP. Once the liver ruptures (starts breaking apart), there is little that can be done to save the patient. A ruptured liver cannot be sewn back together. Sometimes the typical surgical netting is used in an attempt to keep the liver contained. Nonetheless, recovery is unlikely.

High Blood Pressure Medications

Anti-hypertensive medications manage preeclampsia and help avoid eclampsia (high blood pressure plus seizures). Lowering your blood pressure helps prevent strokes and manage preeclampsia. Aldomet is commonly used to help keep blood pressure down during pregnancy, but once you deliver your baby, there are other medication options.

After you deliver your baby, blood pressure can be 130/80 to 140/85 and the effect of hypertensive medications on the baby is no longer an issue (unless breastfeeding). The use of hypertensive medications to keep blood pressures at no more than the postpartum levels of 130/80 will help prevent you from having strokes and damaging other organs. But your pressure must be high enough to supply blood to vital organs.

Commonly used anti-hypertensives include hydralazine and propranolol. Hydralazine has the unwanted side-effect of increasing your heart rate (tachycardia), so propranalol is added to control the heart rate. Generally, these two medications can be started out at low doses and gradually increased upward (titrated) until the blood pressure comes under control. These medications are usually given intravenously (IV) in labor and delivery and by mouth at home.

Take fluctuations in your blood pressure seriously and help your doctor to keep on top of what is often one of the first signs of developing preeclampsia.

NOTES
1. Joelle Goldstein. "'Beloved' Pediatrics Doctor Dies from Postpartum Complications after Giving Birth to First Child." Peoplemag. PEOPLE, November 5, 2020. https://people.com/human-interest/indiana-doctor-dies-from-postpartum-complications-after-giving-birth-first-child/.
2. "Preeclampsia and Pregnancy." ACOG. Accessed March 17, 2023. https://www.acog.org/womens-health/infographics/preeclampsia-and-pregnancy.

CHAPTER 3

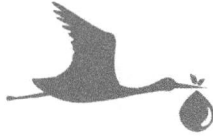

Morning Sickness

Morning sickness is a combination of hypoglycemia (low blood sugar), hypotension (low blood pressure), and motion sickness. In the first three months of your pregnancy, your body has to increase its blood volume by several liters. This increase in blood volume leads to your having low blood pressure part of the time. In addition, your baby will get the blood sugar it needs first, possibly leaving you dizzy and unable to eat.

In the first half of a pregnancy, women are often hypoglycemic (low blood sugar). If you eat a lot of carbohydrates, you will trigger your pancreas to generate a lot of insulin, which will abruptly lower your blood sugar and drive your blood sugar too low. That's when you will have nausea, vomiting, and even become unable to eat.

In the second half of your pregnancy, you are more likely to have high blood sugar (hyperglycemia). You will be able to eat more and not get sick. Your best approach in dealing with both low blood sugar and high blood sugar is diet and exercise. In extreme cases of nausea and inability to eat, you may be given what is called *hyperalimentation*, that is, fluids by IV or NG-tubes, to add fluid and nutrition to your body. This helps your body stabilize your blood sugar levels.

Morning sickness is harder to handle with multiple births. If you are carrying twins or multiples, you will gain about four pounds per month eating the three meals and three snacks suggested to control morning sickness. This is not the time you should be trying to lose weight.

Managing Nausea

Keep crackers and four ounces of fruit juice beside your bed to eat before you get up in the morning. Eat the cracker and juice snack and lie down or sit down for ten to fifteen minutes so the food can settle.

Eat your big breakfast (a second one) before you shower. Eat fat and protein (thirty to forty grams) as well as carbohydrates. Eat bacon, eggs, fruit, and toast. If you are wedded to skim milk and cold cereal for breakfast, as so many of us are, and can't stand the notion of eggs and bacon, try oatmeal. Add butter, whole milk, and a bit of sugar, and have an egg or a slice of unprocessed cheese for protein. Avoid raw cheese to prevent infection with listeria (a dangerous bacterium).

Managing Motion Sickness

Shower *after* your big, second breakfast. The food from breakfast raises your blood sugar and stabilizes your blood pressure.

Avoid driving until you have rested another ten minutes after showering if you don't want to vomit out of your car window. Do not eat in the car.

FIVE WAYS TO REDUCE MORNING SICKNESS

1. Eat like a diabetic
Eat three meals a day with three little meals in between.
All meals should be balanced, including protein (thirty
to forty grams), fat 20 percent, and carbohydrates 30 to
40 percent.

2. Don't avoid carbohydrates completely
This is not the time to go on a low carbohydrate diet.
Rather, aim for 40 percent carbohydrates, 20 percent
fat, and 30 to 40 grams of protein in a meal.

**3. Eat a balanced diet, a diet of three big and three
small meals a day** On a balanced diet, you should gain
two to three pounds a month.

**4. If you find you cannot control the morning sickness
with careful monitoring of your activity and diet, there
are medications available.**
Be aware that while the risks of damage to the baby or
of miscarriage may be absent with these medications,
there are many other side effects of taking them.

Medications for Morning Sickness

Clearly, if you are fortunate enough to be able to control morning
sickness with diet and exercise, you can avoid taking medication to
manage your nausea and vomiting. Of the three commonly prescribed
drugs for morning sickness, studies show they do not produce birth
defects or cause miscarriages, but they all have side effects such as
headache, dizziness, drowsiness, and diarrhea.

ZOFRAN (GENERIC: ONDANSETRON): **Zofran has been considered safe and has been used for years to treat morning sickness. However, Zofran is no longer considered safe in pregnancy. Estimates suggest one out of every four pregnant women receive a prescription for Zofran. Research suggests that while risks appear to be minimal, Zofran should be tried only after all other attempts to control morning sickness have failed.**

REGLAN (generic: metoclopramide): This drug stimulates *peristalsis,* **the muscle contractions which move food through your intestines. While studies indicate there is little risk of major adverse outcomes, studies do indicate it can cause side effects such as dizziness and drowsiness.**

PHENERGEN (generic: promethazine): Phenergen is a Category C drug, meaning it should be given in pregnancy only if the potential benefit outweighs the possible risk to the fetus.

VITAMIN B6 (generic: pyridoxine): Vitamin B6 is said to possibly reduce the severity of morning sickness, but there are risks in those with kidney diseases and malabsorption syndromes.

DICLEGIS: A combination of vitamin B6 and doxylamine, an antihistamine which also aids sleep. The old version of this combination of drugs was called *Bendectin.* **Is no longer manufactured but was popular for decades.**

Vitamins in Pregnancy

Since so much of the control of morning sickness depends upon what and when you eat, this seems as good a time as any to talk about vitamins in pregnancy. Indeed, one of the old tried and true remedies for morning sickness is additional vitamin B6.

During pregnancy, women should take prenatal vitamins, the ones their physicians suggest. You should know what supplements you are taking and why. Talk with your physician about why supplements are important in pregnancy.

My first practice was in a rural Minnesota community surrounded by farms. During the first six months, I had two patients deliver babies with what are called *neural tube defects* (problems with spinal cord nerves). To me, this seemed like a high incidence of this birth defect. At the time, I thought it might be something in the environment. We now know that too little folic acid can cause neural tube defects in the babies of pregnant women. Prenatal vitamins should contain 400 micrograms of folic acid. In fact, the Center for Disease Control and Prevention (CDC) recommends taking 4,000 micrograms of folic acid per day if you have a family history of neural tube defects. You should take 4,000 micrograms a day when trying to get pregnant and continue that level of folic acid intake throughout your pregnancy.

As the American Congress of Obstetricians and Gynecologists (ACOG) notes, the stages of pregnancy where neural tube defects arise is very early in pregnancy. By the time you know you are pregnant, you have passed the stage of pregnancy where neural tube defects develop. So, taking the extra folic acid while you are trying to get pregnant makes sense.

Iron

Iron is also an important supplement to consider when you are pregnant. Your body will make several units of blood during your pregnancy. Because of this increase in the volume of blood, a pregnant woman can appear to be anemic while carrying her baby. Iron is needed to form hemoglobin. It takes about three months for your body to produce red blood cells and for your hemoglobin levels to start increasing after your body's increase in blood volume.

Iron supplements can make you nauseated and constipated, something you don't need in pregnancy. Eat before taking prenatal vitamins. If nausea from oral iron intake is still a problem, talk with your physician. Intravenous (IV) iron is available. Red fruits and vegetables contain iron, which gives them their red color.

You Can Manage Your Morning Sickness

You may have to change your eating habits to help reduce your problems with morning sickness, nausea, and vomiting during pregnancy, but I recommend you try working with your diet to manage morning sickness and nausea during pregnancy before trying to control morning sickness with medications.

CHAPTER 4

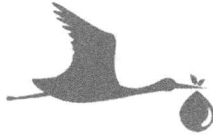

Exercise

Expectant mothers who exercise often wonder about safety during pregnancy. Can they continue their previous regime?

Yes.

However, this isn't the time to try a new routine. As long as the exercise program remains the same as it was before pregnancy, exercise will be safe.

What if your normal exercise routine before pregnancy included strenuous activities such as horseback riding, ice skating, or gymnastics? The issue with any exercise, strenuous or otherwise, is avoiding accidents.

Bike Riding

I recommend against riding a bicycle outdoors during pregnancy because serious injury and death have been known to occur while bike riding on the streets and sidewalks. But a stationary or recumbent bike indoors or in your yard would prevent such accidents. However, once again, let me emphasize to not start new exercise programs during pregnancy. Watch your pulse and keep it under 135.

The motion of peddling will not hurt your baby unless you are having triplets or quads. The real issue is blood supply to your legs while peddling, because some of the increase in blood supply to your legs might be taken from your uterus. So, limit heart rate and the duration to say fifteen to twenty minutes. After your baby is born, you can cycle without limit.

Stopping Exercise

Your baby won't be hurt by stopping your pre-pregnancy exercise program. If you don't feel like continuing your previous routine, you could try cutting back but still exercising a little, if this feels more doable.

Walking Outside

If walking outside is your preferred exercise, you might keep the various seasonal viruses in mind. Outside is a safe place for you to walk, but I would suggest you practice social distancing. There's a lot of disagreement about wearing masks, but I would not recommend a mask if you plan on exercising by walking during pregnancy. A mask will probably interfere with your exercise. It will take more time to get fresh air into your lungs with a mask. You can slow down if this is bothersome. You can also breathe with your mouth open.

Effect of Exercise on Your Baby

Some people fear exercising during pregnancy will cause the baby to be smaller than it would be without exercising. This is not true unless you have started a new exercise program and you are not eating a well-balanced diet, or you are not gaining enough weight.

With Any Exercise Program,
Concentrate on Safety to Your Baby

Whatever your exercise program was before your pregnancy, consider the safety factors to your baby in how you continue to exercise while pregnant. There is no harm done in cutting back on your exercise regimen to be more comfortable during your pregnancy.

CHAPTER 5

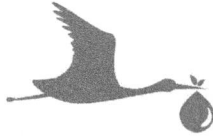

Headaches

In pregnancy, how can you tell which headache is just a nuisance and which one is dangerous? Up to 30 percent of pregnant women are affected by headaches. In general, headaches which precede pregnancy are a nuisance, but benign. On the other hand, headaches occurring after the onset of pregnancy and during pregnancy can be either. Up to 10 percent of patients will have their first headache during pregnancy. The most common kind of dangerous pregnancy headache is caused by changes in blood pressure.

There are about twenty kinds of headaches that can occur during pregnancy and postpartum. The lethal ones are rare, such as headaches which come on suddenly from brain hemorrhage. Another type of lethal headache comes from brain tumors, which develop over time.

I've only seen one patient with a malignant brain tumor in pregnancy. Years ago, during my first year of private practice, I discovered a malignant brain tumor in one of my patients. She presented to the emergency room after a fall. She had new onset clumsiness. Her exam was remarkable for abnormal reflex in her right ankle and knee. A CAT scan demonstrated an astrocytoma. She was sent to a large metropolitan teaching hospital for the duration of her pregnancy.

I never saw her again after her ER visit. I heard she delivered her baby near term but died from her brain tumor four months later.

Hypertension: The Path to Dangerous Headaches

Dangerous headaches are associated with increases in blood pressure. These elevations of blood pressure precede strokes much like going up the steps of a ladder, with opportunity to treat the patient for prevention on each step. The dangerous headaches begin at the foot of the ladder, not once you're on the diving board from the top of the ladder. Know your normal blood pressure and call your doctor immediately if it starts spiking or creeping up and staying up. If your blood pressure goes up even as little as 10 points, you should talk with your doctor.

I've covered high blood pressure, or hypertension, in Chapter 1 of this book. In the case of headaches associated with high blood pressure, I've created a two-step protocol for use with my pregnant patients.

1. Watch carefully for any blood pressure elevation

What appears to be normal blood pressure needs to be watched if it starts spiking or creeping up and staying up. At any time during pregnancy, blood pressure going up and down needs attention. Commonly, blood pressure is checked and rechecked until it starts to come down. However, many women don't know their everyday blood pressure.

Women whose blood pressure goes up even temporarily in pregnancy are a special group who need to be watched closely because it is these women whose pressures will steadily go up and stay up until they develop preeclampsia and possibly eclampsia.

2. Intervene early and gently

With early identification of those likely to become pre-eclamptic, it is easy to begin effective treatment before there is a crisis. I watched my patients' blood pressures closely, so I have not had any patients with episodes of hypertensive crises or eclampsia, and no patients with dangerous headaches, strokes, or seizures.

With early identification of those likely to become preeclamptic, it is easy to begin effective treatment before there is a crisis. Because I watched my patients' blood pressure closely, I had no patients with episodes of hypertensive crises, eclampsia, and no patients with dangerous headaches or strokes.

Those headaches from eclampsia and hypertension are most often from ruptured arteries and are therefore very painful. Some people call them thunderclap headaches because they come on so suddenly. With sudden onset, severe headaches, especially when you are pregnant, you should go immediately to the emergency room and have your doctor called once you are there.

Nuisance Headaches

Most headaches in pregnancy fall under the nuisance category:

- tension,
- migraine,
- cluster, and
- sinus

Tension Headaches

While tension is the most common headache, it is also the most easily treatable. Up to 80 percent of adults get them. Tension headaches hurt all over the head and can feel like a tight headband. Women are twice as likely as men to suffer from tension headaches. Chronic tension headaches can last 30 minutes to seven days. Tension headaches include the following traits:

- start later in the day,
- cause trouble sleeping,
- associated with feeling tired,
- accompanied by irritability,
- make focusing difficult,
- may cause mild sensitivity to light or noise,
- cause muscle aches or a feeling of a tight band around the head and
- are most often triggered by stress.

Unlike migraines, tension headaches won't have other nerve symptoms such as muscle weakness or blurred vision. Tension headaches don't usually cause severe sensitivity to light or noise, stomach pain, nausea, or vomiting. Tylenol has been commonly recommended for pain relief in general, but is now definitely not recommended during pregnancy. I would recommend trying to reduce tension and resting.

Remember, pain medications do not cure tension headaches. Antidepressants, blood pressure medications, and anti-seizure medications are considered better and safer alternatives.

Migraine Headaches

Migraines usually affect one side of the head, the eye, the temple, or the back of the head. Symptoms include:

- no tension,
- visual disturbance or aura before headache onset which brings nausea,
- sensitivity to light and sound, and
- trouble moving or speaking.

When determining what type of headache you have, consider how it feels. Tension headaches are usually mildly painful without throbbing. Migraines come on slowly and increase intensity with physical activity. They often pulse or throb.

Treatment for migraines in pregnancy can be sumatriptan, either oral, injection, or nasal spray. According to The American College of Obstetricians and Gynecologists (ACOG), sumatriptan is the preferred triptan (one of a large class of drugs) because there is the most evidence that it causes no harm and that it is effective.

Comparing Tension and Migraine Headaches

You may be able to determine what kind of headache you have, tension or migraine, by asking yourself two questions.

1. How Often Do I Get Them?

Occurrence varies for both tension headaches and migraines. Tension headaches occur mostly in adult females. Migraines can affect anyone, but men get them more often before puberty and women get them more often after puberty.

2. How Long Do They Last?

Tension headaches can last thirty minutes to up to seven days. Migraines usually last between four and seventy-two hours.

Cluster Headaches

Migraine and tension headaches are the most common headaches in pregnancy, but cluster headaches can occur. These headaches happen in cluster periods or in cyclical patterns. They are the most painful headache. One wakes up in the middle of the night with intense pain in or around one eye or one side of the head. Bouts of cluster headaches can last weeks or months, followed by remission, which can last for weeks, months, or years.

Sinus Headaches

Sinus headaches are most likely associated with sinus infections, tonsillitis, or ear infections. When asked where the pain is, patients usually point to an area above or below their eyes on one side or both. Sinus infections are often associated with runny noses, fever, and chills.

With the effort to reign in antibiotic use, the tendency today is to no longer treat sinus infections with antibiotics. From my experience with sinus infections, I prefer to treat them with antibiotics because sinus headaches don't go away in a week, as colds do. Sinus infections are hard to get rid of, often leading to worse infections in other parts of the body. I have seen a sinus infection spread to the brain. If your doctor says you have a sinus infection, you should ask your doctor to treat the infection with antibiotics. When you're pregnant, your immune system is suppressed, making getting over your sinus infection difficult without antibiotics.

Medications for Headache During Pregnancy

I recommend avoiding Tylenol in pregnancy. If you feel you need some sort of pain medication for your headache, call your doctor.

Most pregnancy headaches are benign, but some aren't. With sudden onset, severe headaches, especially when pregnant, go to an emergency room as soon as possible.

CHAPTER 6

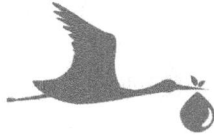

Non-Stress Tests

Obstetricians use a Non-Stress Test (NST) to check on your baby's well-being in the mother's uterus. NST frequency during a pregnancy depends upon the age of the baby in the mother's womb and mother's risk factors, such as diabetes, high blood pressure, or low amniotic fluid. All testing should predict safety or danger. If the test predicts safety, the mother can return home. If the test predicts danger, delivery is indicated.

What is an NST Test?

Tests monitoring fetal well-being have been around for about seventy years. The first test was called an oxytocin challenge test (OCT). This test was like the beginning of an induction with IV Pitocin. Contractions had to last fifty or sixty seconds. They had to occur every three minutes and the fetal heart rate had to be variable, with increases and decreases. When I was a student in the mid-1970s, the nurses would call the OCT an induction, because it often evolved into an induction.

By the time I returned for my residency in 1977, the OCT had been largely replaced by the NST, or an observation of fetal well-being using the electronic contraction and fetal monitors to watch babies' heart rates, variability (short term increases or decreases in rate), and accelerations or decelerations (long term increases or decreases in fetal heart rate). The uterine monitor was used to determine whether there were or were not spontaneous contractions.

A few years later, the fetal kick test, also called a home NST, was developed. All these tests are meant to monitor and predict fetal health by watching babies' heart rates. If the baby passes OCT or the NST, they're considered to be viable for the next three days. So, if there were concerns about the health of the baby, the monitoring occurred every three days or twice a week. The OCT and the NST were expensive and inconvenient.

The expectant mother goes to the hospital or clinic and a fetal monitor is put on the mother's abdominal wall so the baby's heart rate can be monitored and recorded. Another recording monitor is also placed on the mother's abdominal wall to check for uterine contractions. The mother is usually placed on her left side, halfway between lying on her side and lying on her back (the left lateral decubitus position), with the help of a pillow to keep her positioned.

The baby's heart rate should be between 110 and 150 beats per minute, and it should be variable. Flat lines are bad. The variable rate (line) is good, indicating the baby's brain and nerves are intact, with nothing blocking messages coming from the baby's brain going to the baby's heart to keep a normal rate.

A form of fetal distress is a *late deceleration*, or a slowing down of the fetal heart rate after a mother's contraction. This deceleration is caused by the decreasing oxygen supply to the baby from the placenta.

With the evolution of the home fetal kick test, the expense and inconvenience of the OCT or NST were replaced by a home test, which was both convenient and very cost-effective since there was no expense associated with it whatsoever. My patients used this test for years and I found it to be reliable in every way.

How to Do the Kick Test at Home

There are a number of ways to do a kick test, but I have read many studies of various options and the following is my favorite. A half hour after you finish eating lunch (if you eat at 12:30 p.m., do this test from 1:00 to 1:30 p.m.), lie on a comfortable place such as a bed or recliner midway between your left side and your back (the *left decubitus* position). In this position, count your baby's kicks for thirty minutes. There should be ten kicks in the half hour, although some references allow an hour for the accumulation of the ten kicks. If you can feel the baby draw its leg up, that's one kick. Stretching the leg back out is a second kick.

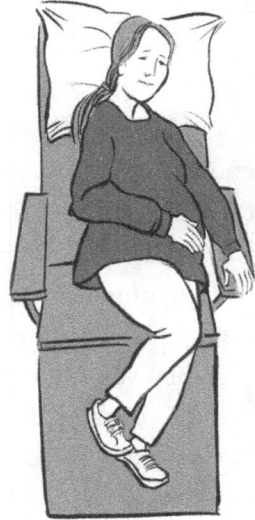

This test is done only once in a day. When to start the kick testing depends upon the age of the baby and what else may be going on with you, such as high blood pressure, diabetes, or low amniotic fluid. If you find that your baby isn't kicking ten times during the test, report your results to your doctor. Your doctor should agree to arrange for an NST test in the hospital or clinic to recheck your results.

Is the Kick Test as Accurate as the NST?

Some studies indicate that the home NST is overly sensitive, indicating distress when there is none. The claim is that the kick test simply causes increased utilization of services and expense. I've found the kick test to be valid, depending on how it is performed, and it is reliable, predictive, valuable, convenient, and inexpensive.

Do All Doctors Use the Kick Test?

Recently, the value of the home NST has been called into question because it has been accused of generating false positive results; that is, indicating your baby is distressed when there really is no distress. Some providers blame the kick test for being false positive (that is, not enough kicks in the half hour), indicating the baby is stressed. When the kick test indicates the baby is stressed, the NST test is ordered to verify the stress. These negative tests, according to the critics, cause further unnecessary testing, which increases cost of the care. My testing has not supported these allegations.

When you go to the hospital for an NST test, you would go to the area of your hospital where babies are delivered (labor and delivery). My patients never had a false negative result from their home kick test that was later shown by a hospital NST that there was no distress to the baby. If you are careful to do the home kick test according to the directions, the results will be accurate, either positive or negative.

When Your Baby Kicks Frantically

You need to be aware that often babies will move frantically just before they die. If you experience this kind of movement, go to the labor and delivery department of your hospital right away. If you are sent home dismissively, I recommended you call your doctor or go to a different hospital. Your concerns should not be dismissed.

Spend some time learning to do a kick test successfully and you will have a safe, inexpensive way to follow your concerns about your baby's well-being.

CHAPTER 7

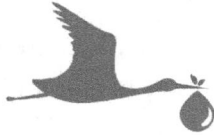

Hormones

There is a dance-like play of hormones that work throughout your pregnancy, delivery, and postpartum to choreograph your safe and healthy delivery of a newborn baby. With so much intervention in today's labor and with inductions of various kinds, with some knowledge of the role various hormones play in your labor and delivery, you have a better understanding of what happens with hormones in natural labor and delivery as opposed to how the hormone cascade plays out in various kinds of inductions.

In order to proceed properly in labor, the emotional brain needs to dominate our newer, higher brain, our rational brain. This diminished consciousness is induced by beta endorphins and is inhibited by bright light, loud noises, conversation, and fear. It's no wonder that labor sometimes slows or stops by coming to the hospital. For millions of years, this hormone cascade has been actively and effectively causing natural labor, milk letdown, and decreasing anxiety with the net result that mothers are better prepared to take care of their babies and to negotiate their postpartum course.

For years, those of us trained in obstetrics have listened to moms and dads or significant others come to labor and delivery with the announcement that they are in labor. Once in the labor and delivery unit, labor stops. We were trained to think that you and your husband or SO simply don't know what real labor is. I've come to believe that many of you really were in labor, but became anxious or even afraid when you arrived at the hospital. You are immediately bombarded with bright lights, loud noises, people milling around, cold rooms and cold bedding, pelvic exams, and IVs. Fear and anxiety stopped your labor. Laboring women respond best with one or two familiar and friendly faces and a warm, dark, and quiet room.

Years ago, we observed women in the labor and delivery unit for a few hours, assuring their health and safety, and then put them to sleep with 15 mg of morphine IM and 200 mg of Seconal IM. Laboring mothers did very well with this approach, and many of them actually woke up completely dilated, having slept through their entire labor.

Today we have many reasons (most of them not good) to avoid these medications. Nobody died from those medications, neither the mothers nor the babies. The idea was to give enough of the medication to achieve the desired results, which it did.

Estriol and Progesterone

During the acceleration phase of labor (when the cervix dilates from 5 cm to completely open), beta-endorphins induce a feeling of well-being and diminished consciousness. Estriol and progesterone are the hormones that set the stage for labor. Both are produced by the placenta. Progesterone has a ten- to eighteen-fold increase in pregnancy. Found in only small amounts in the non-pregnant woman, estriol from the placenta surges to 1,000 times what it was at the onset of labor. Estriol increases the number of oxytocin receptors and muscle cell connections in the maternal uterus late in pregnancy, preparing the coordination of uterine contractions in labor. Together the beta endorphins—the progesterone and the estriol—activate pain relieving pathways in the brain and spinal cord.

Oxytocin

Oxytocin is made in the hypothalamus and stored in the posterior (back part) of your pituitary gland. The pituitary gland releases oxytocin impulses every three to five minutes to promote effective contractions, especially in your acceleration phase of labor. Oxytocin is nature's form of Pitocin, a powerful contraction-causing hormone released during sexual activity, orgasm, birth, and breastfeeding.

After your baby is born, eye-to-eye and skin-to-skin contact stimulate the release of oxytocin. Oxytocin is present in your brain and switches on your mothering instincts. In addition, oxytocin stimulates your sense of smell, further releasing oxytocin and promoting mothering. Oxytocin suppresses your adrenal gland, making you sleepier during pregnancy, which, if you think about it, conserves your energy. It also helps to keep breastfeeding mothers more relaxed and more resistant to stress.

Prostaglandins

Prostaglandins are also an important part of labor and delivery. These hormones initiate prodromal (pre-labor softening and thinning of the cervix) active labor and continue stimulating labor during the remaining natural labor. They are found in high levels in semen, and they are responsible for orgasm, uterine contractions, and period pain. These prostaglandins are potent and set the stage for oxytocin release in the acceleration phase of labor.

Endorphins

Endorphins are a naturally occurring opiate similar to morphine. They are very important in pain suppression and creating a sense of well-being with decreasing awareness, which is also part of normal labor. In addition, endorphins activate dopamine, increasing feelings of well-being. In the breastfeeding mother's brains and cerebrospinal fluid, endorphins take more than twenty hours to break down, and therefore are long lasting. They also act to suppress your immune system so you can tolerate the presence of a your baby, who is only 50 percent your DNA.

Epinephrine and Norepinephrine

Epinephrine and norepinephrine are produced in response to stressors such as hunger, cold, fear, loud noises, bright light, starting an IV, pelvic exams, and excitement. They stimulate the fight or flight system. Rising levels of these hormones in early labor can inhibit your uterine contractions, slowing or stopping labor. Norepinephrine reduces blood flow to your uterus, your placenta, and your baby.

Natural labor provides the hormone cascade which is beneficial to you and your baby. This cascade can be promoted by warmth, quiet, darkness, and the presence of familiar people like a husband or a midwife.

CHAPTER 8

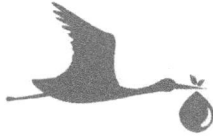

Stress and Anxiety

Anxiety is the most common psychiatric disorder. Women are twice as likely as men to be diagnosed with it. If you historically suffer from anxiety, you are likely to need strategies to deal with it and keep you and your baby happy and healthy during and after your pregnancy. Onset of new anxiety during pregnancy is common. Please communicate with your doctor if this is your experience so you can get additional support as needed.

Journaling helps promote self-esteem and is an excellent technique to help you manage your anxiety and depression at home. If you have not already started your journal, please consider doing so. You may go over your journal yourself. That's therapeutic. Or you may share your journal with your physician. Take three or four of the concerns you have journaled about, write them down, and share them with your provider. Your physician may suggest you see a counselor. If you get a referral to a counselor from your physician, don't be shy about seeking help.

Does My Anxiety Create Risk to My Pregnancy?

Anxiety and other stresses in pregnancy are associated with miscarriage, preterm delivery, and delivery complications. If you are suffering from anxiety and become pregnant, it's important to work with your doctor to create an action plan so you can optimize your pregnancy outcomes. Journaling can be a big part of the action plan.

Some Natural (drug-free) Ways to Deal with Anxiety During Pregnancy

Enlist the help of your partner in creating and maintaining a calm pregnancy environment. You can also try yoga, meditation, and walking. Be sure to talk to your obstetrician, as well. If your obstetrician doesn't feel comfortable helping you with your anxiety, ask for a referral to a counselor.

Is it Safe to Take Anxiety Medications While Pregnant?

Taking anxiety medications during pregnancy does carry some risks to your baby (depending upon the medication) including cleft lip and "floppy baby syndrome" (hypothermia, lethargy, poor respiratory effort, and feeding problems). Your infant may also suffer from withdrawal from certain medications. Be sure to consult with your prescribing physician and understand all the risks before making your decision.

Whether to take or not to take antidepressants during pregnancy is a complex decision. Bottom line: if you need them, take them. The benefits of taking antidepressants during pregnancy will almost certainly outweigh the risks of not taking the medications. Sometimes in pregnancy you have to make a choice between risk factors.

What if I'm on Anxiety Medication When I Get Pregnant?

Work with your prescribing physician. Your choice depends on what medications you are taking and how much you need them. One option is to slowly decrease your dosage over a period of about three weeks until you can wean yourself off of your medication. Another option is to switch to a different anti-anxiety medication, and still another option is to keep taking your present medication and dose. This is a discussion you need to have with your physician.

In the end, you have to consider three possibilities:

1. The benefit of taking the medication.
2. The risk of taking the medication.
3. The risk of NOT taking the medication.

In the end, the decision needs to be weighed from the perspective of where the greatest benefit will be compared to the greatest harm. If not taking your medication could result in self-harm, for example, your physician may recommend that you continue taking your medication in spite of the potential risks to your pregnancy. The decision as to which path to follow is yours to make with input from your physician.

SECTION 3

You Can Adjust Your Flight Plan for the Unexpected

We've talked about the kinds of things obstetricians watch during your pregnancy. We have encouraged you to talk with your physician about the choices you have in your pregnancy so you can choose the care you feel works best for you.

But there are a few unexpected events which can turn up on the way to delivering your baby. Your plans for these events should be added to your flight plan:

- multiple births,
- genetic factors,
- ectopic pregnancy,
- miscarriage, and
- premature birth.

In any flight plan, unexpected events occur which will require adjusting your course. Your flight plan is flexible. You can add or subtract information as your pregnancy progresses. Discuss the unexpected with your physician and amend your flight plan with the choices you prefer.

CHAPTER 9

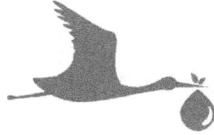

Multiple Births

Jean, at twenty-six years old, presented to my office with her husband, Dan, after two years of infertility. My nurse placed her in an exam room and took her vitals (blood pressure, heart rate, and temperature).

"Nice to meet you, I'm Dr. Alan Lindemann" I said. "I hear you would like to get pregnant."

In any initial fertility visit, one of the first questions a doctor asks is, "Have you been sexually active?"

Jean responded, "Yes, we have been married for two years, but my periods are somewhat irregular. I have about seven periods each year."

I continued reviewing her medical history. "I see the rest of your history is normal. Your mother had three children without any difficulty, Is that correct?"

"Yes, I have two brothers who are younger than I am," Jean answered.

"I would like to do a physical exam now if that's okay with you."

I listened to her heart and lungs. They were fine. Jean had no abdominal masses. Her pelvic exam was normal and her pap test from six months earlier was also normal.

"Since there is no purpose to treating your wife for infertility if you are infertile, I will order a semen check."

Dan agreed, and the semen check came back normal. With the normal semen check, I told Jean "I will start you on Clomid to help you to ovulate."

I prescribed Clomid at 50 mg by mouth once a day for days five through nine of Jean's next menstrual cycle.

Jean returned to see me in three months. She was about six weeks pregnant. Initially, her pregnancy went well. Her labs and physical exams were normal. At about twenty weeks, her blood pressure began to increase and reached 125/80. By twenty-four weeks, her pressure had risen to 140/90. Clearly she was pre-eclamptic. An ultrasound of her baby indicated it was not living. Jean spontaneously delivered her stillborn baby shortly after her visit.

Jean returned to my office a week after her delivery. She returned again in four weeks. She seemed to be successfully grieving. The examination was normal, including her blood pressure, which was now 110/70.

Jean wanted to become pregnant again and asked for more Clomid. We had a long discussion about the risks and benefits. I prescribed more Clomid. Three months passed; Jean returned to my office, pregnant once again. On examination her uterus was large for gestational age. I did an ultrasound exam and could see three babies.

I was worried. This young woman with preeclampsia and hypertension had barely passed the midpoint of her pregnancy with one baby. Could she carry three babies long enough for these babies to be able to survive at birth?

"Jean, you are carrying triplets. They are all living at this time. We need to talk about your maintaining this pregnancy until you reach at least thirty-three weeks with these babies. Please stop smoking. For the time being, I'm asking you to work six hours a day, not eight, and certainly not twelve. You will need to take it easy and rest, but I do not recommend bedrest, as bedrest has no proven benefits and increases risks for blood clots and strokes.

"Please buy a blood pressure cuff. A medium price cuff is probably best for you to use at home. It will offer you better performance than a cheap one and lacks the unnecessary trappings of the most expensive cuffs. Check your blood pressure twice a day. Once in the morning about 8:00 a.m. and again in the evening about 8:00 p.m. If either your top or bottom number goes up ten points, call me right away."

I continued my recommendations for Jean to increase the safety of her pregnancy and delivery with her triplets. "I'm going to ask you to gain about four pounds a month. If you have trouble eating, let me know. I want to see you every week in the clinic so I can keep an eye on your blood pressure, your urine protein, and your reflexes."

Jean came to my office every week for her prenatal visits. Her blood pressure remained good until she reached thirty-four weeks. At that time, her pressure rose to 135/85 and she went into spontaneous labor. By reaching thirty-four weeks, she had carried the babies long enough for them to live once they were born. I delivered three healthy baby boys, each weighing about 3.5 pounds, each by C-section. The babies were small but did well after birth.

Several decades later, I was working on call in a hospital emergency room when a police officer brought in a patient. When I read his name tag, I recognized him immediately as one of the triplets I had delivered so many years before.

There are numerous stories of women thinking they were carrying only one baby, only to be surprised at delivery with a second baby. Today, with ultrasound, this is unlikely to happen. An ultrasound at twenty weeks will identify multiple births.

All multiple pregnancies require an increased level of care and attention from both the mothers and their doctors. You should see your doctor more often than if you were carrying only one baby. If you know you are carrying twins or triplets, be sure to ask your doctor how often you will be scheduled for prenatal visits compared to women carrying only one baby. It's important to protect your health and your babies' health during pregnancy, delivery, and especially during their first few months of life.

Stay in touch with your care provider through each step of your journey, and don't hesitate to ask these and other questions to help you incorporate the information into your unique pregnancy and birthing experience.

Giving birth to multiples offers more risks for problems in your pregnancy. But in my experience, it's not twice as much risk.

Multiples are more common with in-vitro pregnancies. Some fertility physicians refuse to deliver multiples from in-vitro fertilization. The parents of the quadruplets I delivered came to see me because they did not want to allow selective reduction of the number of babies from four to two. You may learn more about their story in my interview of the quadruplets when they were twenty-one years old.[1]

In all my years of obstetrical practice, I've delivered four batches of triplets, all born alive and healthy.

Delivery

In most cases, it is possible to deliver twins without a cesarean section, and even without an episiotomy (surgical cut made at the opening of the vagina). In my first practice, fresh out of residency, I delivered four sets of twins in my first six months of practice.

Your obstetrician needs to discuss your options for delivery with twins or multiple births. If your twins are both head-down, you need to ask your obstetrician his or her comfort level with managing your delivery. Today, many obstetricians prefer to deliver twins and even breech babies (feet or buttocks positioned to come out first instead of the head) by C-section. When I was in residency, we were taught how to deliver breech babies and twins without C-sections. So it's not unreasonable to ask your doctor to deliver your twins vaginally.

If you're expecting twins, you may be wondering if there are certain considerations you need to be aware of that are different than when you are carrying only one baby. In my experience, about 50 percent of twins are both head-down in the uterus. The next most common presentation is first baby is head down and second baby is feet down. The second baby can be delivered breech or turned by external cephalic version (ECV). With ECV, your doctor turns the feet-first baby by externally manipulating your stomach to change the baby's position. Either option is reasonable. Twins can also both be breech, and I have delivered twins vaginally when both were breech. It can be done and with good outcomes.

Of these four possible presentations, if both babies are head to head, that is the first baby breech with feet first and the second baby head down, this is considered a poor choice for a vaginal birth because of the chance of the babies locking chins. The pregnant women I've treated have not exhibited this presentation, but the ACOG recommends a C-section in such cases.

So in most cases, yes, it is possible to deliver twins without a C-section, and even without an episiotomy. However, you may find yourself in a situation where your first twin is delivered vaginally and the second one by C-section. In my opinion, this is the worst of both worlds. Management of the second twin requires patience, discernment, judgment, and luck. Of these, patience is the most important. A new mom who has a combination vaginal/C-section delivery with twins will be more tired and sore; she will need much support at home to avoid depression. Recovery time will also be longer, from four to six weeks.

To avoid the vaginal/C-section combination delivery, women need to know their options and discuss them with their doctor. If your babies are not both head-down, what is your obstetrician's comfort level with managing the delivery? If your obstetrician is adamant that the babies must be delivered by C-section, ask for a recommendation for a consult with an obstetrician willing to deliver twins vaginally. You could also ask members of a "mother of twins" group for their recommendation for an obstetrician willing to deliver twins vaginally.

Sometimes twins are born on different days. I've done enough deliveries that I have had one twin deliver on one side of midnight and the other on the other side of midnight. Actually, I have had twins deliver on separate days, separate months, and even separate years (New Year's Eve/New Year's Day)! I'm not sure what the parents did about birthday parties or schools. Ironically, I later moved to a small town where I discovered my neighbor across the street happened to be the grandmother of the twins I delivered in two separate years.

Major Concerns by Trimester

When carrying twins, nausea, lack of interest in food (anorexia), and risk of miscarriage are high in the first trimester. In the second trimester, risk of preterm cervical dilation and hypertension are greater than for a single baby. You will probably delivery your twins at around thirty-eight weeks. This is considered "term" for twins.

In my first practice, a lady presented to my office carrying twins. She had been a neonatal intensive care nurse in Boston before moving to a small town about fifty miles from my clinic. Her cervix was thin and had dilated to 1 cm at twenty weeks. I was worried, but I recommended she go home, avoid strenuous activities, check her vitals, return in two months, and call me with any questions. She returned in two months and there was no cervical change. She continued checking her blood pressure and vitals and returned at thirty-six weeks. She still had no change in her blood pressure or her cervix. She delivered healthy twin boys vaginally at thirty-nine weeks.

Nursing Twins

Nursing twins can be done. Most often, nursing is simultaneous with each baby getting a breast. Nursing is wonderfully adaptive. The babies can be held like a football under each arm, with the head on the breast and the body and legs to the mother's sides and back.

Most importantly, don't worry! About the only thing that wrecks nursing is worrying and thinking you can't. If you think it can't happen, it won't.

Until your milk production catches up, you may need to top off your twins' feedings with formula. Please do not worry when providing your twins with some supplemental formula. Your babies need to eat and gain weight. They should double their weight by six months and triple their weight by twelve months.

Exercise

Maintaining your pre-pregnancy exercise program depends upon what your pre-pregnancy program was. If you were not running one mile a day before you got pregnant, I would avoid running one mile a day while you are pregnant. The rule of thumb is no new exercise regimen during pregnancy. Yoga would be a better choice than new exercises in pregnancy. Swimming is a good choice, but stay out of public pools and stay out of hot tubs because of high temperature and growth of bacteria.

Diet and Eating

Although we know the optimum weight gain for singleton pregnancies, less is known about multiples. My experience with twins indicates you should eat about 40 percent more than with single pregnancies, but not twice as much. You need an absolute amount of protein, not a percentage. If you are carrying one baby, I recommend 130 grams of protein per day in six meals. For twins, you will need another 20 or 30 grams of protein per day. With twins, you need to eat enough to produce more amniotic fluid, more placenta, and more baby than in a singleton pregnancy.

Postpartum Depression

A multiple pregnancy can have everything a single pregnancy can have, but more of it. So yes, more baby blues, more depression, and for some, the increased possibility for post-partum psychosis. See Section 6 in this book on postpartum depression. Years ago, no one paid much attention to postpartum depression, but thankfully, more is known about it now and you no longer have to have guilt feelings about how you feel about your new baby.

Dads can play a big part in postpartum support. In my experience, dads attending prenatal visits and classes are much more able and willing to help out after delivery. Be sure to welcome your partner to all your prenatal visits. The father of the quads I delivered took an active part in caring for his babies. He told me he changed 7,000 diapers per month! Now that's dedication and commitment!

Set your mind at ease by learning more about what it means to carry, birth, and raise twins or triplets. The more knowledge you have, the more you will be able to advocate for yourself with your care providers and navigate all the unique realities that having twins will present to you.

CHAPTER 10

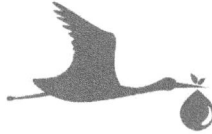

Genetic Factors

Sherry, a recently married twenty-six-year-old on oral contraceptives, presented to the emergency room with chest pain high on the right side of her back. I always taught my medical students that they needed to ask the right questions of their patients to get the information they needed to decide on the correct diagnosis.

"Do you have any increased pain when you breathe?" I asked her.

"No," she responded.

I continued to try to get some notion of what was going on with the pain in her back. "How about shortness of breath?" I asked.

"No," again.

I rephrased my question. "Do you have pain in your legs or shortness of breath when you are walking up the stairs?"

"No pain in my legs, but I am short of breath when I go up a flight of steps," she admitted.

With that response, I highly suspected a pulmonary embolism (blood clot in lung). Finally, I was beginning to find the correct question to ask.

"Sherry we're going to order a CAT (computerized axial tomography) scan with dye (angiogram) of your lungs to look for pulmonary emboli," I explained.

The results of Sherry's angiogram were remarkable. The angiogram showed many pulmonary emboli in her lungs. This is not something you expect to find in a young woman Sherry's age.

"Your angiogram shows multiple pulmonary emboli. I want to refer you to Fargo for treatment," I explained to Sherry. "They could at least remove some of the many blood clots in your lungs, if they think it's necessary."

The problem with pulmonary emboli in the lungs is that they prevent the lungs from functioning properly and you could die from lack of oxygen. The physician I referred Sherry to shared with me that she would have died with any more pulmonary emboli.

With this many pulmonary emboli in so young a woman, I tested Sherry for the genetic factor methylenetetrahydrofolate reductase deficiency (MTHFR). The current medical stance is to not only not test for MTHFR, but not treat it when it is found in a patient. In North Dakota, 40 percent of the population carries some form of the MTFHR. I had no problem ordering a test to check Sherry for this genetic factor despite the current medical position on not doing so. In this case, Sherry's test results showed she had a particularly aggressive form of MTFHR.

She was initially treated with Lovenox and then switched to Coumadin, a medication she will probably have to take her entire life.

With treatment for her MTHFR, Sherry was able to go back to college and became a med tech. So, this discovery not only saved her life, but also actually changed it a lot. But I had to ask the right question to hone in on Sherry's MTFHR.

Autosomal Disorders

If this is your first pregnancy, you should look into the ways genetic factors can affect your baby. Some genetic factors may be surprises, and some you may know are part of your family history. For example, you may know from family history that you carry the gene for Tay-Sachs or Huntington's Chorea. But there are other factors which you may be unaware of unless you have problems with them in pregnancy. Generally, women know to watch for Rh negative blood with pregnancy. However, there are a number of other genetic factors which can be involved in pregnancy outcomes. Factor V Leiden (FVL) is one. Cystic Fibrosis is one. Another is an enzyme, methylenetetrahydrofolate reductase (MTHFR).

I consider attention to the following recessive genetic factors important for a safe and successful pregnancy:

- Rh negative blood,

- clotting disorders, and

- autosomal recessive disorders.

RH Negative Blood

While genetic testing is something obstetricians are sometimes told to avoid for fear of false positives, the test for your lack of the Rhesus factor in your blood is not one of them. In other words, every single pregnant woman should be tested for the Rhesus factor. Rhesus factor is a place on the red cell which carries oxygen in the blood from the lungs and delivers the oxygen to the body cells. It is an autosomal (body chromosome as opposed to a sex chromosome) dominant gene. You either have the Rhesus factor or you don't. You are called Rh positive if you have the Rhesus factor and you are called Rh negative if you do not have the Rhesus factor.

If you are Rh negative and your baby's father is Rh positive, it is likely that your baby will be Rh positive. If your baby has the Rhesus factor and you do not, there is the likelihood that a little bit of your baby's blood will leak into your bloodstream. It takes only a few milliliters (there are 30 milliliters in one ounce) to sensitize you to make antibodies against these foreign Rh positive cells coming from your baby. During subsequent pregnancies, your permanent antibodies will cross through your blood, your placenta, and into your baby and destroy your baby's hemoglobin, causing anemia. With low hemoglobin (anemia), your baby may be unable to survive, or at best, will be born prematurely.

Treatment of Rh Negative Women with RhoGAM

Years ago, before we understood the Rh factor or how to prevent problems for a mother and her baby, the first baby of an Rh-negative mother would most likely be born alive. Subsequent babies would be stillborn at six months or less. Every pregnancy loss would be earlier because the antibodies would increase. My mother had a brother who married an Rh negative women. Back in the 1950s, I can remember the sadness that we all felt over their pregnancy losses. Before RhoGAM, Rh negative women lost baby after baby to the antibodies building up in their blood with every pregnancy.

After RhoGAM began to be used, there was a time when moms and dads were both tested for the Rhesus factor. If the fathers were Rh negative, there was the idea that there was no reason to give RhoGAM. Today we have come face-to-face with the difficult truth that the baby's dad sometimes isn't the husband. Therefore, RhoGAM is now given to Rh negative mothers without testing the fathers.

When I was in residency, we gave RhoGAM to Rh negative mothers after their babies were born. In the mid 1980s, we began following the Canadian practice of giving RhoGAM in the late second trimester, at about twenty-seven to twenty-nine weeks. RhoGAM works by tricking your body into thinking that your own antibodies are not needed because the Rh antibodies delivered by RhoGAM are present, but these antibodies are only present temporarily. Since the mother is not creating the antibodies supplied in the RhoGAM, the RhoGAM antibodies eventually become weaker and disappear. Giving a pregnant woman RhoGAM before the baby is born avoids the potential for Rh sensitization to the baby. However, the RhoGAM may be waning in its effectiveness by the time you deliver your baby. For this reason, you should get another shot of RhoGAM within three days after your baby is born.

The three-day window for giving RhoGAM originated in the RhoGAM studies done in the early 1960s with prisoners. The subjects were injected with RhoGAM on Friday and their blood tested on Monday. There was really no scientific investigation to warrant the three-day limit. It was just a matter of convenience. The three-day window was effective, and without testing this time period, we still use it as the standard for providing RhoGAM to Rh negative mothers with Rh positive babies.

RhoGAM Needed Even for Miscarriages

It is very important that RhoGAM be given at the time of a miscarriage because just a small amount of Rh factor in the blood is all that it takes to sensitize Rh negative mothers. The dose for miscarriages is less than the dose given during or after pregnancies. But if you get the big dose for your miscarriage it won't hurt you. Better safe than sorry. RhoGAM is also indicated for spotting, external cephalic version (ECV), amniocentesis, or other procedures where blood exchange between the Rh negative mother and her baby could take place.

Cystic Fibrosis

Cystic fibrosis is so common, ACOG recommends that all patients who are considering pregnancy or who are already pregnant should be offered carrier screening for cystic fibrosis regardless of ethnicity. The CDC has also added cystic fibrosis screening to newborns. With cystic fibrosis, there is a wide range of clinical severity. Average life span is thirty-seven years, which is much longer than it used to be. Approximately 15 percent of babies born with cystic fibrosis have a milder disease and can survive longer. Negative screening does not eliminate the possibility of having cystic fibrosis because of the possibility of having uncommon mutations. When I was growing up, a family in the community had nine children. All were born with cystic fibrosis and all but one died at a young age.

Cystic fibrosis is an autosomal recessive gene, meaning the gene must be in both parents, not just one parent. Screening, however, significantly reduces the risk. If both parents are carriers, chorionic villus sampling or amniocentesis can determine whether the baby has inherited one or both of the parental mutations. Prognosis is based on the degree of pulmonary disease. Since this disorder is autosomal recessive, in theory only one of four children would have an active form of the disease, two would be carriers like the parents, and one would have no gene for cystic fibrosis.

Genetic counseling is challenging because the cystic fibrosis gene can manifest in a significant variety of severities. If you would like genetic counselling, ask your doctor for referral.

Tay-Sachs Disease

This is an autosomal recessive disorder which requires the recessive gene from each parent for the baby to develop Tay-Sachs. As with cystic fibrosis, another autosomal recessive factor, if the couple have four children, the affected offspring has two doses, one from each parent, two children will be carriers, like the parents, and one child who is neither a carrier nor affected by it, with no dose of abnormal genetic material. Risk for Tay-Sachs would be one in four children would have the disease. It is possible for any couple to have two, three, or even four children who are affected by Tay-Sachs or four children who have no illness at all. Each child has a one in four risk of having the disease. Risk is for each child and is not based upon the number of children you have.

The disease is characterized by an enzyme absence causing progressive degeneration of nerve tissue and death in early childhood. At risk groups include Ashkenazi Jews of Eastern European, French Canadians, or those of Cajun descent. ACOG recommends screening should be offered before pregnancy if both members of a couple are Ashkenazi Jewish, French-Canadian, or of Cajun descent, or if there is a family history of Tay-Sachs disease.

Clotting Disorders

Clotting disorders include genetic conditions such as Factor 5 Leiden (FVL) and methylenetetrahydrofolate reductase (MTHFR). It's not fashionable now to screen for MTHFR. However, in my area, 40 percent of the population carry some version of MTHFR. If you know you have a family history of clotting disorders, be sure to tell your doctor. Have any of your parents died in their thirties from a heart attack or stroke? Has anyone in your family had a deep vein thrombosis (DVT)? With a family history of clotting disorders, your physician should check your risk for them early in pregnancy and work with you to treat them! Your doctor should also check for clotting disorders if you have had several miscarriages or suffer from infertility.

Factor V Leiden (FVL)

Having Factor V Leiden (FVL) increases your tendency to form blood clots in your blood vessels. In pregnancy, this gene increases the risk of developing a deep vein thrombosis (DVT) seven-fold. If you have FVL, you will probably be given anticoagulants (such as Lovenox) during your pregnancy to prevent miscarriage and to prevent DVTs while carrying your baby. Besides DVTs, with FVL, there is a slight increase in the risk of the loss of your pregnancy.

MTHFR

Recently the declaration has come down from on high in medical practice that no one should be routinely tested for MTHFR. Labs have stopped testing for MTHFR. I regard this as short-sightedness largely promoted by insurance companies who want to save money by not paying for services some may need. As mentioned, I practice in an area where about 40 percent of the population has some form of MTHFR. Furthermore, I have seen what kinds of problems can be caused in pregnancy by the more serious of the three gene variations labeled MTHFR.

I have seen women with repetitive miscarriages who, when they are diagnosed and treated with Lovenox, carry their pregnancies to term every time. So, because of my personal experience with MTHFR, I'm reluctant to tell anyone to forget about it. Sometimes even milder forms seem to present with increasing cardiovascular problems, like strokes, pulmonary emboli, deep vein thrombosis (DVT) and heart attacks as described in this chapter's introductory story about Sherry.

MTHFR is also associated with neural tube defects in babies. It is often recommended that folic acid be taken to prevent neural tube defects, which includes spinal bifida. If you have some forms of

MTHFR, your body is unable to use vitamin B12 effectively, which your body requires to produce folic acid, which prevents neural tube defects such as spina bifida and anencephaly (lack of a brain).

ACOG says that neural tube development occurs in pregnancy so early that women do not know they are pregnant. Therefore, testing for MTHFR during a prenatal visit to prevent neural tube problems would be too late to be of any use. ACOG recommends taking 400 mcg folic acid a month BEFORE planning to get pregnant.

In my practice, I have seen two patients with neurotube defects. In one case, I did an ultrasound at fifteen weeks because of *polyhydramnios*, a condition in which there is too much amniotic fluid. This ultrasound indicated there was a neural tube defect (NTD). There are differing degrees of NTDs. The defect can occur from the head to the tailbone, with the outcome better the lower the NTD occurs in the spine. The tail bone NTD has the best prognosis. This patient's baby had her NTD by her tailbone, so her prognosis was good. When my patient reached thirty-nine weeks, I scheduled her for a C-section. Mother and baby did well.

Years later, a patient came to me for an ultrasound, which demonstrated hydrocephaly (fluid taking the place of brain tissue), another result of neural tube problems in pregnancy. Of the two NTDs, anencephaly and hydrocephaly, hydrocephaly has the potential for a better outcome for the baby. She wanted no destructive procedure. She chose to continue the pregnancy. No evacuation of the fluid on the baby's brain. We planned for a C-section when she went into labor. As it turned out, she presented to my office in labor. While in the waiting room, I heard her scream and we quickly got her into an exam room. Her water broke, the baby presented breech, and the baby was delivered shortly afterward. Eight years later the patient called me from Chicago to tell me her little girl had lived for eight years.

Contrary to the current medical practice to not test for MTHFR in pregnancy, I have seen too many problems associated with this genetic condition to recommend not testing for it. Ideally, you should know about whether or not you have an MTHFR gene variation BEFORE you become pregnant. You can then be sure you are taking methylated vitamin B12 before you become pregnant. Share your concerns about MTHFR with your doctor, preferably before you become pregnant.

Autosomal Dominant Disorders

Children are born with forty-six chromosomes, or twenty-three pairs. One of the twenty-three pairs comes from the mother and one of the twenty-three pairs from the father. In the mid-1800s, Gregor Mendel, an Austrian monk, studied single traits associated with gene pairs. His findings indicated that a single trait could be dependent upon whether one of the genes in a pair was dominant or recessive. Brown eyes, for example, can result from one of the two genes for eye color to be brown, which is dominant. The gene for the eye color blue, on the other hand, is recessive, meaning to have blue eyes, both of the genes in the pair for eye color need to be blue.

With autosomal recessive disorders, two genes with the disorder need to be present in the child for the condition to develop. Prenatal screening for genetic problems in pregnancy is now much less invasive than it once was. Introduced in 2012, prenatal (first trimester) screening with cell-free DNA became available, and testing can now be done with a maternal blood draw. This has significantly reduced the number of invasive prenatal diagnostic procedures. There has been a 70 percent decline in early placenta sampling (CVS). There has been a nearly 50 percent drop in amniocentesis procedures following the introduction of cell-free DNA screening.

If you know you have a family history of genetic disorders, you may want to ask your physician for a referral for genetic counselling.

Huntington's Chorea

This is an autosomal dominant condition, meaning only one gene on one chromosome is required for the disease to manifest itself. With dominant chromosomal diseases, a child has a 50/50 chance of carrying the Huntington's gene. Huntington's is characterized by jerky, uncoordinated movements, progressive dementia, and psychiatric symptoms. The mean age of onset is forty years, so prenatal care often ignores this genetic factor because the late onset of the disease is far in the future and therefore does not complicate most pregnancies. Prenatal screening is controversial. Extensive counseling is important because of the late onset of the disease. If you know the Huntington's gene is in your family history, I would advise you to request your doctor to text you before you are pregnant and refer you to genetic counselling if you find you are carrying the gene for Huntington's.

Other Autosomal Dominant Disorders

There are many autosomal dominant disorders. Marfan Syndrome and the BRCA1 and BRCA2 genes are two that are fairly well known. There is a 50/50 chance of passing on an autosomal dominant disorder to your children. If you have any concerns about your family history, talk with your doctor about them. If you would like genetic counselling, ask your doctor for a referral.

Genetic Counselling

The field of genetic counseling has grown as our knowledge of DNA has developed. Years ago, amniocentesis was often used to test for genetic problems. Today, blood tests can be used instead of amniocentesis to sample your own or your partner's genetic makeup. With this information, you can make decisions about the possible outcomes your and your partner's genetic factors may have on your baby. However, sometimes genetic conditions depend upon more than one gene pair. There are numerous genetic conditions which may affect your pregnancy. Discuss any of your concerns with your doctor and do not hesitate to ask your physician for a referral to a genetic counsellor.

CHAPTER 11

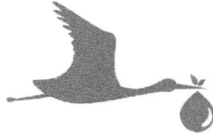

Ectopic Pregnancy

Alisha came to my office concerned about her IUD and pelvic pain. She said, "I've had my IUD for six months, but now I have pelvic pain and I feel pregnant."

Upon examination, I couldn't find the IUD string, and her ultrasound showed no intrauterine pregnancy and no IUD in her uterus. Yet her pregnancy test was positive.

"Alisha," I explained, "I need to do a laparoscopy to look for your pregnancy and your IUD. When did you eat last?"

With the laparoscopic surgery, I could see the tubal pregnancy near the end of her right tube. That was fortunate, because that is the easiest place to remove an ectopic and still keep her tube intact. I was able to remove the ectopic and easily control the bleeding. But finding the IUD was more difficult. I knew it was there because I could see it on the x-ray of Alisha's abdomen.

Eventually, I found the IUD. The IUD had gone completely through Alisha's uterus, through her small bowel, and had gotten stuck in her large bowel. Remnants of these layers of uterus and bowel were stuck on the IUD. I pulled out the IUD and called our surgeon to over-sew the bowel to prevent leaking bowel fluid. Alisha did well, but she was done with IUDs after that.

I had not placed this IUD. When IUDs are inserted poorly by the physician, many problems can develop. This is one reason we have a string on IUDs.

Yes, perforation is one complication of an IUD. Although this seldom happens, the perforation is usually just through the uterus and not through several layers of bowel as well. It is amazing that Alisha didn't get into more trouble with all the bowel perforations.

In an ectopic pregnancy, the fertilized egg grows outside the uterus, usually in the fallopian tube. Most ectopic pregnancies are tubal, but the fertilized egg can implant on the ovaries or any other organ within your stomach cavity. The pain from ectopic pregnancies usually starts on either the right or left lower quadrant. Initially, the pain is from stretching of the fallopian tube, but eventually the pain may become excruciating from bleeding into the abdomen.

By the time many women end up in the emergency room with abdominal pain, they have no idea that they're pregnant because they have mistaken the bleeding from an ectopic pregnancy for bleeding from menstruation. Remember that blood loss from your bleeding ectopic can be significant; as many as several units of blood. Once the blood reaches your diaphragm in the upper part of your abdomen, you will have shoulder pain on one or both sides. Shoulder pain is a late finding and means you need to be getting to the emergency room.

Women with ectopic pregnancies usually present to the physician with the second episode of bleeding. They often have mistaken the first episode of bleeding as a period. The examining physician needs to ask the right question, that is, "When was the last normal period?"

Usually, ectopic bleeding would be lighter than a normal period. With ectopic pregnancies, abnormal bleeding may start around seven weeks after the last normal menstrual period. When presented with a patient with a possible ectopic pregnancy, physicians need to ask a woman when her last NORMAL period occurred. There is bleeding when an ectopic pregnancy implants, and this bleeding can often be confused for a period.

In the United States, surgery has been the standard of care for ectopic pregnancies, but there are some countries in which methotrexate is the standard treatment rather than surgery. Methotrexate works over time, and that time may vary from patient to patient. Whether methotrexate can be used to treat an ectopic pregnancy depends upon the patient's level of human chorionic gonadotropin (hCG), ultrasound findings, and the amount of bleeding, so sometimes surgery is still the best option.

Surgical treatment resolves a pregnancy that can't be saved immediately. If you go to the emergency room (ER) with an ectopic pregnancy, you might simply be given methotrexate and sent home. Being sent home with methotrexate may require several return visits to the ER. This will become more expensive, dangerous, and time consuming than surgically removing the ectopic pregnancy. If you find yourself in the ER with an ectopic pregnancy and you want surgical treatment, say so.

Survival from ectopic pregnancies is much better today than we have seen previously. Advances in the quality of ultrasound have improved women's outcomes. The advances in measuring the level of hCG have also increased the ability to diagnose ectopic pregnancies accurately and early.

CHAPTER 12

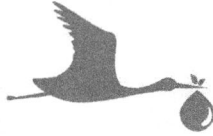

Miscarriage

Miscarriage is defined as pregnancy loss prior to twenty weeks. If the pregnancy lasts beyond twenty weeks, but is unsuccessful, it is termed stillbirth.

Who can have miscarriages? Anyone. The most often quoted numbers are 10 to 20 percent of all pregnancies end in miscarriage. Now, with new pregnancy tests and ultrasound, pregnancy can be diagnosed before the first missed period. When the miscarriage rate includes those fetuses lost before the missed period, the miscarriage rate increases to 40 percent.

Miscarriage is quite common, yet regardless of that simple truth, it remains a challenging and emotionally complex experience for women. It is often something women cope with privately with their partner.

"It was the worst day of my life," Kay told me. "I was lying on the exam table and the technician was looking and looking at the ultrasound image. She said nothing. Just continued to study the image. Finally, I asked her if that wasn't two babies I saw, and she said, "yes." I knew then for the first time that I was carrying twins. But something was wrong and that technician wasn't talking about it except to ask, "Are you sure when you got pregnant?""

A friend of Kay's had recommended she come to see me because she wasn't getting answers from her regular obstetrician.

"I had been to my regular obstetrician's office four weeks earlier for my previous prenatal checkup," Kay continued, "the doctor hadn't been able to hear a heartbeat even though I was fifteen weeks pregnant. He assured me that wasn't so unusual and asked me to wait four weeks to do an ultrasound."

The next visit went no better, Kay continued. "So, four weeks later and nineteen weeks pregnant, as I lay on the doctor's exam table looking at the ultrasound image, I learned for the first time that I was carrying twins—and that they were dead. I had been carrying my dead twins for four weeks." Kay added finally, "They were boys."

It's unusual for a pregnant woman to carry dead babies as long as Kay had. That is why I always treated miscarriage actively instead of letting my patients carry dead babies indefinitely.

Kay continued her story of a doctor who didn't really care much about being sure she got the care she needed. "Even though I lived in a rural area forty miles from a hospital, the doctor sent me home with no instructions about what to look for or what to do."

The only instruction I got was the doctor's comment, "You will eventually lose them at home."

Kay told me how upset she was at how the doctor handled her situation. "I went home devastated. I was afraid I had done something to lose my babies. I've always taken good care of myself when I was pregnant, eating carefully and being cautious to avoid exposing myself or my babies to anything harmful." But, Kay added, "I had two little girls already and perhaps I hadn't been resting. I agonized over what I could possibly have done to lose my twins."

Many of my patients drove long distances to see me and I often didn't know how they had heard of me. In Kay's case, she lived near the town I first practiced after my residency. In any case, she told me, "When I got home, I called your office and made an appointment. To my surprise, I was given an appointment the very next day. I had to travel over 140 miles round trip to see you, but I was just glad to be able to see you so soon."

Linda, my ultrasound tech, looked at that image for less than one minute and said these were identical twins developing from one amniotic sac. Linda told Kay, "When twins develop from one amniotic sac, sometimes their umbilical cords get tangled and the twins are unable to survive."

Later, Kay told me, "That simple statement let me know that I hadn't done anything to harm my twins."

After Linda had completed Kay's ultrasound exam, I entered Kay's examination room and looked briefly at the ultrasound. As gently as possible, I let her know that these babies had not died because of something she had done. I needed to try to deflect the guilt I knew she felt with her miscarriage. I knew this was the beginning of successful grieving with noticeable, observable, tangible loss. I knew my ultrasound tech had told her about the problem, but I wanted to let her know I agreed with what my ultrasound tech had told her. "Your twins have not developed a separating membrane to keep their umbilical cords from getting tangled," I said.

I knew Kay lived far away and would not have time to get to a hospital when she began to deliver these dead babies. I asked Kay "How long has it been since you ate last? I want to schedule your dilation and curettage (D&C) surgery as soon as possible."

I was able to schedule her for that evening at 8 p.m.

Kay came to my office for her follow-up appointment a week later. She had created a keepsake box for her twins. She told me, "We had a memorial service for our sons, Benjamin and Joshua, and our minister held a short service at the grave site when they were buried. My husband and I felt it was important to name our twins and honor them."

"Both my husband and I wrote letters about the twins and put them in their memory box. Letters from relatives and friends are also in the box. Our daughters added notes and art, as well," she added.

Kay was able to talk about how helpful the memory box was in working through her and her family's grief. "This has been a tremendous help for all of us and has allowed us to honor and respect the memory of our twins."

Kay's story is a good example of successful grieving with tangible loss.

Pregnant with twins at twenty weeks, Kay and her husband presented to my office knowing Kay was carrying dead twins. Kay's previous obstetrician hadn't detected heartbeats at fifteen weeks. A month later he did a sonogram and told her that the babies were dead, but that he would run some hormone level tests. In the meantime, he told Kay to go home and wait to miscarry. She lived forty miles from the nearest hospital, but she was still sent home without any instructions for what to watch for if bleeding problems developed.

All miscarriages need to be managed actively. When patients leave the office, they need to understand the difference between normal and abnormal miscarriages. With a normal, early miscarriage at about seven weeks, you will have about one day of heavy bleeding. Bleeding will be heavier than a normal period, but less than one soaked super-pad per hour. If, like Kay, you are carrying dead babies with no sign that spontaneous delivery will occur soon, then your doctor needs to define limits for you. You cannot carry dead babies indefinitely. You need a plan to define how long you wait at home for a spontaneous miscarriage and plan for a D&C once you've exceeded the defined wait time for spontaneous delivery.

Normally I try to offer as much choice as possible to my patients who miscarry, but I was concerned that the denial of Kay's previous provider had narrowed the length of time we could wait for the D&C. Kay had already lost a lot of choice because her obstetrician had spent so much time in denial. To promote successful grieving, I knew it was important to deal definitively with the death of her twins, not only for Kay's physical safety, but also for her mental health.

While discussing our options, Kay told me she would be okay if she could see the babies and take them home to be buried. We talked about how to get the babies so she and her husband could take them to their funeral director. I told them that the nurses would take the babies away during the procedure, but I would retrieve them, even though I knew the nurses would object to this change in the hospital routine.

All tissue removed in operating procedures is placed into formalin and taken to the lab. I did the D&C. While Kay was still under anesthesia, I rescued the babies from the formalin and put them in a plastic bag. I gave the babies to Kay's husband in the waiting room. I admitted Kay to the hospital overnight because she lived so far away and I had done the D&C so late in the day. Admitting Kay to the hospital was the right thing to do because she experienced heavy vaginal bleeding in the night. The nurses were successful in stopping the bleeding without much difficulty.

The next morning, I was paged by the hospital CEO, a man I seldom saw. He demanded an explanation for my giving the twins to Kay and her husband because they wanted to have a funeral and bury them in the cemetery. That's the way they had chosen to grieve. The CEO accused me of stealing tissue for some nefarious purpose. He then asked me why I did things in the hospital which he considered outside of the norm. He complained that my actions were irresponsible and that it would take several days and lots of phone calls to straighten out this mess. He claimed I had violated federal law and that I had brought trouble to the hospital.

I called Kay and her husband asking them to verify that I had given the "tissue" to them. They called their mortician. He called me right back and said he was sorry for this hassle. He needed only a transportation permit. He signed and faxed it to me. I signed it, faxed it to the mortician, and then sent him the original. Everything was legal and done with one signature. There indeed was nothing nefarious. It's too bad there are so many people who are so interested in making healthcare decisions so difficult when they could be made so easily.

Kay and her husband returned a week later for a routine post-operative visit and I had the chance to check the progress of their grieving. I was thankful that I could see that Kay and her husband were adjusting. They felt they were on the right track with their grieving. They had achieved the closure they had wanted. They chose to have normal, successful grieving for a tangible loss.

Six months later, Kay was back in my office newly pregnant. This time only twenty-five days into the pregnancy, I could see Kay was again carrying twins and that each one had its own amniotic sac.

Miscarriage or Stillbirth?

Miscarriage before there is a beating heart is common and is usually a chromosomal mutation which doesn't support life. These are not preventable. However, once the heart is beating, several conditions can lead to a miscarriage.

Repeated miscarriages often *can be* preventable. If you have had two miscarriages, it's time to look at the list of treatable conditions that are known to contribute to miscarriage in some women (for example,

Strep B, social disease, or blood clotting problems).

With a Doppler, I can hear a heartbeat at about eleven or twelve weeks. However, it is easier to *see* the heartbeat with an ultrasound at seven to eight weeks. If I can't see the heartbeat at seven or eight weeks, out of reverence and concern for the baby and the mother, I recheck again in one week. If I can't see a heartbeat, even on the second check, I discuss miscarriage. Many women prefer to wait for a spontaneous miscarriage.

Spontaneous miscarriage usually follows one or two weeks after discovering no heartbeat. If one or two weeks go by without a miscarriage, I recommend misoprostol (Cytotec) by mouth. While it is possible to use misoprostol without waiting the two weeks for a spontaneous miscarriage, it would not be my first choice because aggressive treatment can interfere with the grieving process. I prefer to allow a wide margin around guilt, blame, shame, and depression.

Miscarriage is traumatic for all pregnant women and their partners. If you have had, are having, or will have a miscarriage, remember this:

Miscarriage is NOT your fault.

I always suggest waiting for at least one regular period before getting pregnant again. That way your new due date can be more accurately determined. In addition, having a normal period signals your body is done with the miscarriage process.

Grieving for Your Loss

I consider the most important part of a miscarriage the grieving process. I have often said that I could only handle three miscarriages in one week. With each pregnancy loss, my emotional batteries are drained a little bit more. It is impossible to participate in another person's grieving sequence and not be affected by it. When physicians are not affected by the grieving processes of their patients, it is time for them to find a new career.

One precaution: *always remember that after a miscarriage, getting pregnant again can be easy.* Some doctors say wait for three months before getting pregnant again. I always suggest waiting for one regular period before getting pregnant again.

CHAPTER 13

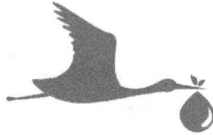

Infertility and Recurring Pregnancy Loss

Claudia and Matthew were schoolteachers who had made a career of teaching English as a foreign language in many other cultures and on many continents. They were in my office for an ongoing infertility evaluation and treatment. They had undergone significant workups on other continents and three rounds of in vitro fertilization without success.

"I've never been pregnant," Claudia said.

Matthew added, "We're only here for ten days before we go back to Japan."

Claudia's and Matthew's physical exams were normal. I did my usual cultures for Group B, chlamydia, gonorrhea, aerobes, anaerobes, ureaplasma, and mycoplasma.

"Claudia, you test positive for ureaplasma," I reported after the test results came back. "I've found that this organism often causes no problems with getting pregnant, but for some women, it does. I'm going to give you both prescriptions for doxycycline."

Three months later I got a call from Claudia in Japan. Claudia was pregnant for the first time.

Seven months later they called again. Claudia had delivered a healthy, eight-pound baby girl with good Apgars.

Sometimes the most expensive treatment fails when the least expensive treatment succeeds. The official stance on the bacteria ureaplasma and mycoplasma are that these organisms are so common in everyone that they are not considered to be pathogens (organisms which cause illness). Instead, they are considered to be what we call colonizers (organisms which don't cause illness). They are present in your system, but cause no harm.

In my practice I have found that for some people, common organisms can cause infertility, as ureaplasma had for Claudia and Matthew. These same organisms could also cause miscarriage or premature birth. Recently, the notion has surfaced that these common bacteria can indeed cause much harm, not only for infertility, but also for pregnancy loss. It will probably be decades before ureaplasma and mycoplasma, for example, are commonly recognized as possible problems for couples who have infertility problems or repeated miscarriages.

When you become pregnant, you're not thinking about miscarriage, pregnancy problems, preeclampsia, preterm birth, or stillbirths. But the unfortunate truth is that up to 10 percent of women will have some kind of problem during their pregnancy they may not have anticipated.

Recurrent pregnancy loss from preterm birth is not always handled well by our current healthcare system. Many women suffer from two or three pregnancy losses before anyone will take their losses seriously. In my practice, I found being able to take a woman with recurrent pregnancy loss through a successful pregnancy and delivery of a live newborn was remarkably fulfilling.

The largest cause of neonatal mortality is preterm birth. Commonly, we most often say there is no reason or explanation. So rather than saying, "I don't know," I said to myself, "Let's look and see if we can find something we can change that will give you a living, healthy newborn baby."

In working with women who had had recurrent stillbirths, I found several topics that are not commonly considered with recurrent pregnancy loss.

Fibroids

Most doctors will agree that recurrent mid-trimester pregnancy loss due to fibroids (benign smooth muscle tumors) is treatable and preventable. I agree. Fibroids can be found in various intrauterine places. If they remain in the wall of the uterus and do not encroach on the uterine cavity, most of the times they don't cause any serious problem. They can cause cramping during pregnancy, but they are generally not associated with preterm or stillbirth.

When the fibroid encroaches on the endometrial cavity, where the baby will be, or if the placenta attaches on or near the fibroid, there are problems. Fibroids are easily removed by a variety of procedures that are safe and effective.

Placental Abruption

Placental abruption, or separation of the placenta from the wall of the uterus, is associated with bleeding, prematurity, having had many pregnancies, advanced maternal age, and uterine scars (such as from a C-section). If I had a patient with placental abruption who lived more than fifteen minutes from the hospital, I placed them in a non-hospital room for $15 a day. The floor with these non-hospital rooms was directly below the labor and delivery floor. This provided safety for my patients so they were actually in the hospital if their abruption needed immediate attention. Nurses were nearby if needed. Everybody there did well with what I referred to as the "hospital hotel."

With placental abruption, sometimes there's a little bit of bleeding in the second trimester, but that often stops. However, if the bleeding doesn't stop and the mother's hemoglobin decreases, the treatment for placental abruption is delivery. Unfortunately, delivery of the baby at thirty weeks isn't always the best option for the baby. If you are close to term, you do not necessarily have to have a C-section as long as you are not bleeding and your baby is not in fetal distress.

Placental abruption is a common cause of preterm birth, but it does not seem to be recurrent. The reasons for placental abruption don't necessarily change; in other words, you're still probably going to have a history of having many children, advanced maternal age, or some kind of uterine scar, but you will not necessarily have a second pregnancy with placenta abruption.

Group B Strep

Group B as a source of recurrent preterm delivery and stillbirth is not commonly understood in the practice of obstetrics. I know that sooner or later somebody from the ACOG will read this and they'll probably be upset, because according to their understanding of Strep B infections, the organism does not ascend up the vagina and into the uterus. Rather, ACOG believes this infection comes from the gastrointestinal tract and moves across the skin between the anus and the vulva (perineum) and into the vagina, and I agree with this. However, group B strep is not supposed to cross through the cervix, the upper part of vagina, the amniotic sac, the placenta, the amniotic fluid, and into the baby. But in the 6,000 babies I have delivered, I had no maternal or neonatal mortality from group B strep because I treated my patients early for group B strep, and repeated treatment if it returned before delivery of the baby.

I have observed only one baby sick with group B. The common lore is that babies delivered by C-section won't be infected with group B strep because they do not pass through the birth canal. I was asked to do a C-section for another physician. This was a repeat C-section of a mother who did not have ruptured membranes and was not in labor. Yet upon delivery, it was clear her baby had been very sick in utero with group B. Luckily, the baby had a very good neonatologist who diagnosed the problem right away and treated the baby successfully and the Strep B did not recur.

If the baby is not sick upon delivery from group B strep, exposure to group B strep by passing through the birth canal of a mother with group B strep opens up the possibility that the baby can develop infection later. Usually the first sign of infection is pneumonia at birth or meningitis at three months. Physicians will possibly tell parents of babies hospitalized for pneumonia at three months from group B strep that the baby will not get sick again from the infection. However, I know of a baby who had pneumonia, the first infection with group B, and had the meningitis infection from group B a few months later. The baby was not supposed to have group B twice, but he did indeed have pneumonia and then three months later meningitis.

Many studies of group B consider it not to be an ascending infection. I believe this is a misconception. I have always cultured group B early in my patients on their first or second prenatal visits because I believe strep B is indeed an ascending infection. The organism is capable of moving up the vagina and into the uterus. When collecting cultures, it's important to collect samples from your vulva, not just the top of the vagina. With only samples from the top of the vagina, any strep B in your vulva would be missed and your culture could be negative even though the group B strep could be on your vulva.

I also learned early in my practice to culture and treat for group B strep in patients who have recurrent pregnancy loss and infertility. ACOG considers group B strep a common organism in women and believes that even if they treated for it early in a pregnancy, it will just reappear before delivery. When my patients had group B strep, I treated both the mother and father for group B strep, and if it reappeared, I treated both mother and father again. That way my patients could go into labor and not have to rely upon being given IV antibiotics for group B strep during labor.

Ureaplasma and Mycoplasma

ACOG and I also disagree on the treatment of the ureaplasma and mycoplasma during pregnancy. ACOG believes these organisms are not pathogenic and that ureaplasma in particular is a common colonizer in our bodies. There are many different kinds of ureaplasma, and we cannot determine which kind is present based upon the average ureaplasma culture. I also believe there are many women who go through pregnancy with ureaplasma and have no problems. However, those who cannot go through pregnancy without problems from ureaplasma deserve effective treatment so they can carry and deliver a healthy baby.

My particular group of patients with a history of recurrent pregnancy loss or infertility would get tested for ureaplasma and mycoplasma, be treated, and then often go on to get pregnant, and stay pregnant long enough to deliver a healthy baby. I had a very large infertility practice based upon this unorthodox notion.

Chlamydia and Gonorrhea

There is no doubt that chlamydia and gonorrhea are considered to be pathogens. They commonly cause infertility by making scar tissue in and around the fallopian tubes and even sometimes in the uterus. More serious complications for these pathogens would be an abscess in the fallopian tube and sometimes between the tube and the ovary.

Chlamydia is now the most common sexually transmitted disease (STD). I generally routinely checked my prenatal patients for chlamydia and gonorrhea, along with the other organisms discussed in this chapter.

Syphilis

Syphilis is very uncommon today, but is still tested routinely in prenatal care. Until fifteen or twenty years ago, silver nitrate was placed in a baby's eyes on the chance that the baby might have been exposed to syphilis. More recently, instead of placing silver nitrate drops in newborn eyes, a thin ribbon of erythromycin ointment is placed on the baby's eyelids.

My experience with infertility, miscarriage, and recurring pregnancy loss has shown me that as obstetricians, we need to be much more attentive to many kinds of common colonizing bacteria early in pregnancy. In the current medical environment, getting the attention you need early on for these conditions may be one of the your most challenging prenatal tasks, especially if you have had recurrent pregnancy losses.

SECTION 4

Deciding Where to Deliver Your Baby

During my OB/GYN residency back in 1977, we were taught that home births with midwives were bad and hospital births with physicians were good. While an increasing number of women are electing to have their babies at home despite this OB/GYN position, we in the profession need to ask ourselves why women would choose a home birth.

Part of the answer can be traced back to the principles of informed consent. You have the right to disagree or choose to turn down the healthcare your physician offers. You have the option of signing or not signing the informed consent form. Your doctor has the obligation to treat you even if you do not choose the treatment option your doctor prefers. If your doctor decides to not treat you because of your choice, your doctor has an obligation to refer to you another doctor. Today, these elements of choice are significantly lacking or compromised in typical clinic-based and hospital-based care. And yes, lack of autonomy bothers some women so much so that they opt for home births.

Deciding whether you want a hospital delivery or a home birth is one of your most important decisions in your pregnancy. You need to explore your options early in your pregnancy, even as early as interviewing and selecting which physician seems to work best with you. Even as early as this first visit, you might start a list of the pros and cons of home birth versus hospital birth in your Flight Plan. Continue to add to this list as your pregnancy progresses.

I have learned over the last forty-five years that hospital births are not necessarily the best, safe, or good and that home births are not necessarily risky or bad. What matters is who does the delivery, where your delivery will be done, and how your delivery will be done.

CHAPTER 14

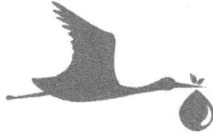

Choosing a Hospital or a Home Birth

As you mull over your decision as to where to have your baby, you should ask yourself whether you would feel more comfortable giving birth at home or in the hospital. Did you know that anxiety can interfere with labor? It is not uncommon for labor to stop for a while when you check into a hospital for delivery. If labor stops for any length of time, your obstetrician may suggest induction to speed things up.

I have always tried to manage patient anxiety by promoting confidence and comfort in my patients within the hospital, giving them the autonomy and respect they would have at home. The big problem with hospital births is the loss of autonomy, which starts with your insurance company telling you which doctor you may see and which hospital you may go to. Furthermore, you will get a predefined number of visits and tests, with insurance companies continually trying to cut costs by decreasing the number of paid-for visits and the length of your stay in the hospital. In hospitals, the insurance company's clock rules the time of your baby's birth.

If you want a delivery with the least amount of technological intervention, you will probably need to work with a midwife and have a home birth or find a birthing center rather than a hospital. Many people feel that birth is a natural process and should be allowed to progress without a lot of technological intervention. Midwives usually see their patients more often than physicians. However, many insurance companies do not cover the services of midwives.

There are some serious health conditions you may encounter during your pregnancy and birth that might push your decision about where to have your baby towards the hospital instead of a home birth. But for many, home birth provides a reasonable alternative to hospital birth.[1]

In a hospital, even with a "normal" delivery, you will probably have an IV (medications given directly into one of your veins). There will likely be external monitors, and sometimes internal monitors tracking your contractions and your baby's heart rate, and a blood pressure machine. You might have a Foley catheter for collection of your urine because you are tied to the bed with monitoring equipment and can't easily get out of bed to go to the bathroom. Walking is good for a natural labor, but when you are in the hospital hooked up to numerous pieces of electronic equipment, arranging to walk around to help your delivery is difficult.

In the hospital, the fetal monitor is supposed to make birth safer for babies, but all it has done is increase the C-section rate. The fetal monitor strips are often hard to interpret and can easily be misread as indicating fetal distress, resulting in emergency C-sections. Remember, during your initial interview with your obstetrician, you asked what his or her C-section rate was. You also asked at this time what the C-section rate was at the hospital. There is tremendous variation in the number of C-sections from hospital to hospital. If you opt for a hospital delivery, you want a hospital and an obstetrician with a low C-section rate. All this information you collected in your Flight Plan will be handy when you are trying to make your decision about whether you want a hospital or home birth.

In the Scandinavian countries, many deliveries are done at home and the health professionals all work together and maintain good communication. Women in these countries also enjoy one of the lowest maternal mortality rates of industrialized nations, with only two to three maternal mortalities per 100,000 births. In these countries, the mother chooses where she wants to deliver her baby: at home, in a birthing center, or in the hospital. Midwives work cooperatively with doctors to provide frequent visits and comprehensive oversight of patients.

In some areas, you may have an option of a birthing center designed to provide a more home-like environment to deliver your baby. Birthing centers aren't hospitals, but they have a working relationship with hospitals in case of emergencies.[2]

From my perspective, we need to create specialty birthing hospitals with an operating room so there is the hospital safety net, nurses, doctors combined with the autonomy, comfort, voluntariness, and respect that mothers would get with a midwife at a home birth or birthing center. Ideally, the labor, delivery, recovery, and postpartum should actually be like home, not just give the appearance of home with pretty drapes and fancy wall coverings.

Unlike other medical specialties, obstetrics allows your doctor or midwife to work together with you to bring new life into the world. Though not everything can be controlled during pregnancy, you still have many opportunities to choose the kind of labor and delivery you prefer. Choosing where to deliver your baby is one of those choices, one that will have a profound effect on everything about your labor and delivery.

NOTES

1. L. McClurg, (2019, March 11). "Home birth can be appealing, but how safe is it? NPR. Retrieved February 6, 2023, from https://www.npr.org/sections/health-shots/2019/03/11/700829719/home-birth-can-be-appealing-but-how-safe-is-it.

2. Contributing Writer/Editor Maressa Brown, "Delivering at a Birth Center," What to Expect, December 15, 2022, https://www.whattoexpect.com/pregnancy/birth-center/.

CHAPTER 15

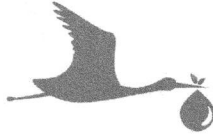

Natural Birth

Joan was carrying twins when she came to see me.

"Nice to meet you, Joan. Did someone refer you?" I asked.

"Yes, Jackie recommended you," she said. "I feel a little big and am concerned about having twins. They run in my family. My last period was seven weeks ago."

"Let's get an ultrasound exam," I responded. "You have two living babies here, at seven weeks," I reported.

Joan's pregnancy went along well, with twelve prenatal visits and normal labs, growth, weight gain, and vitals, but at thirty-five weeks both twins were breech. Even with the breech twins, Joan asked, "I want to have a vaginal birth. Can I?"

I said, "I don't see why not. You've delivered your first baby vaginally. Your first baby weighed ten and a half pounds. We'll do a double set up. I mean we'll be ready to do a C-section delivery if we need to."

Sometimes breech babies will turn into the usual head first position by the time they are ready to be born. However, these twins were still breech when they were full term.

Her pelvis was certainly proven. These twins were her

second pregnancy. With twins, thirty-nine weeks is considered term. Joan was at thirty-nine weeks and five days. Her cervix was soft and thin and ready for delivery. We started an oxytocin induction. With her cervix ready for delivery, I knew an oxytocin IV induction would work well.

The secret to a successful vaginal breech birth is to keep the baby's head bent forward, chin on chest. This is the reason we have been told to **NOT** pull on a breech baby's feet. Pulling on the baby's feet causes the baby's head and neck to stretch. In my experience, keeping the head supported with pressure on the mother's uterus works well. Often one can get a finger into the baby's mouth to make sure the baby remains looking posteriorly, towards mom's back. All these actions cause the smallest head circumference to enter the mother's birth canal. If the baby's neck is extended, the largest circumference of the baby's head presents to the mother's pelvic inlet, making the baby undeliverable and resulting in a failed vaginal breech birth.

Joan's delivery was done in the old delivery room, which had been converted into an operating room. The anesthetist was present and C-section instruments ready to go if needed. I let the buttocks of the first baby deliver to the umbilical cord, then I brought out the legs, then the arms, and then made sure the baby's face was directed toward Joan's back (sacrum). Lastly, my right hand controlled the baby's mouth and with the left hand I placed pressure on the mother's bladder to keep the baby's head flexed. The first twin was born with better than usual Apgar scores.

I found the feet of the second twin, and keeping this twin's neck flexed, pulled the feet down, then the arms, and I once again placed pressure over Jane's bladder to keep the baby's chin flexed against the baby's chest. The second twin delivered with equally good Apgar scores.

If a labor and delivery is allowed to occur without technological interventions, there occurs what I call a *hormone cascade*. The activation of these hormones in your labor and delivery cause progressive intensity of uterine contractions and pain relief. The cascade starts with prostaglandin from the placenta. Later, your body adds oxytocin, then prolactin, endorphins, and even epinephrine. These hormones cause labor to progress while adding natural pain relief, a feeling of well-being, and getting you ready for birth and breast feeding. The oxytocin also helps uterine contraction after birth, preventing hemorrhage.

In my experience, mothers like a dark, warm, quiet, and safe environment for delivery. They should be able to choose who is present, such as a significant other and a doula. Common activities which interfere with the hormone cascade include bright lights, loud noises, a cold environment, starting an IV, and all of the other testing which mothers get when hospitalized during labor. Fear causes the release of epinephrine and norepinephrine out of sync with the natural hormone cascade, and this increases anxiety, suppresses labor, and interferes with the baby's heart rate. In natural labor, the hormone cascade begins with your body's natural production of oxytocin after five centimeters of cervical dilation. How oxytocin interferes with the natural hormone cascade depends upon when it is introduced.

The first half of labor is about getting ready to deliver. Prostaglandin is released. This softens the cervix and vagina, softening and opening the pelvic joints as the baby's head descends. In an induction, adding oxytocin before 5 to 6 cm of cervical dilation increases pain and creates the need for an epidural. Since nature adds oxytocin in the last half of delivery and labor, the early introduction of oxytocin in labor induction creates intense contractions earlier in the labor than would occur naturally. Oxytocin creates what are called *pit pains*.

Pit pains

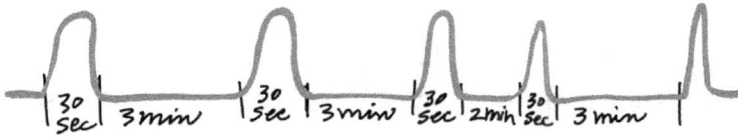

30 sec | 3 min | 30 sec | 3 min | 30 sec | 2 min | 30 sec | 3 min

Induced labor with pitosin

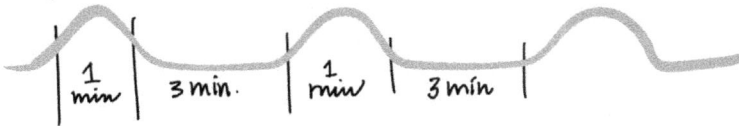

1 min | 3 min. | 1 min | 3 min

Natural labor

The induction contractions spike painfully and do not last as long as natural labor contractions, which grow slowly in intensity and subside slowly.

With natural labor, your hormone cascade will create what I call your "Zen world." The hormone cascade prepares and augments your movement into an altered state of consciousness, which in turn relieves some of the pain of labor. The most important addition to your labor is your body's pain-reliever, called endorphin. This is your body's own morphine. Endorphin puts you in a state of altered consciousness and is, for example, the primary driver in the performance of many athletes.

The hormone cascade described here prepares you for bonding, increases your feeling of well-being, promotes uterine contractions, and decreases the risk for postpartum hemorrhage. It also increases your awareness of smell and touch, which augments breastfeeding.

While it is impossible to say exactly how the introduction of synthetic oxytocin before 5 to 6 cm dilation will influence your labor, the truth is that it most likely does. Natural oxytocin added by your body to the second half of your labor with your prolactin, endorphins, and epinephrine create your hormone cascade. There are no research studies indicating how an epidural affects your hormone cascade during labor and delivery, including how synthetic oxytocin affects endorphins, prolactin, oxytocin, and bonding instinct.

If you want a natural labor and delivery, talk with your doctor during your prenatal visits. You might also talk to the nurses in the hospital labor and delivery unit to see how willing they are to discuss birthing options with you. You might go to prenatal classes and ask if any of your classmates are interested in natural birth. If they are, they might be willing to share with you any success they have had in locating a supportive environment for natural birth.

CHAPTER 16

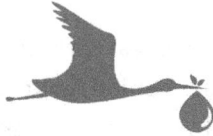

Cervical Ripening Leading to Labor

Geena came to my office with her husband, Paul. Geena was forty weeks and three days pregnant according to her last period and her ultrasound. Her baby's growth, vitals, and weight gain had been normal. Fetal movement had been normal. She had come to my office on this day for cervical ripening with Cytotec.

"Good Morning," I said. "Nice to see you both. Do either of you have any questions about what we'll be doing today and what we will attempt to accomplish?"

Paul said, "You've explained this in detail over the last several weeks. You will place a small dose of Cytotec (25 mcg) in Geena's vagina and wait for early labor."

"Yes, we are looking for the preparatory phase in labor called the prodromal portion, when small, short contractions will appear on the external uterine contraction monitor. We'll also watch your baby's heart rate to be sure it's normal. We'll expect to see small and frequent contractions along with some cervical effacement (thinning), and your baby's head descend into the pelvic area. So, in addition to watching for the presence of frequent little contractions, we'll be looking for contractions which are too strong," I explained.

I continued, "I'm glad you brought along some food. We have fruit and juices, toast, crackers, and water available if you want. I'll leave the room, Geena, and you may get ready, please."

I returned in five minutes with 25 mcg of Cytotec. "I'll place this 25-mcg dose behind your cervix in your vagina. That's it. We're done for now. I'll take you to one of our small private labor rooms, where my nurse will put on your monitors and we'll watch you for several hours to establish enough, but not too much labor."

We checked in on Geena every fifteen minutes.

After four hours, Geena had passed the frequent little contraction part of prodromal labor and gone into a later, more established pattern of contractions. The baby's heart rate showed no distress. Contractions were still not very painful, and Geena was ready to go home with Paul for a while.

Four hours later, I got a call from the hospital delivery unit. Geena came in 6 cm dilated, 90 percent effaced, her bag intact, and with a reactive baby with no fetal distress. Thirty minutes later when I arrived, Geena was in active labor. Geena delivered an 8 lb 8 oz baby boy with good Apgars and with no epidural, no episiotomy, and with NO postpartum hemorrhage.

Prodromal labor is the first stage of labor, where the fetal head descends into the birth canal, the cervix thins and softens, and your baby's head begins to move in position for labor. This stage of labor usually takes the form of a backache or possibly menstrual pain and is dominated by your body's production of prostaglandin.

Cytotec Used in Two Different Ways

The medicine Cytotec is used in two different ways in labor and delivery. It can be used for what is called *cervical ripening*, which prepares the cervix for labor and delivery. Or it can be used for induction of labor. If your doctor is going to use Cytotec in your delivery, you need to know which of the two ways your doctor is using the medication, so you know what to expect.

There are various kinds of prostaglandins (a hormone-like lipid) used for cervical ripening. If a cervix is favorable; that is, showing signs of getting ready for delivery, small amounts of Cytotec or its generic form, *misoprostal*, can promote the process of your cervix getting ready for delivery. I would place 25 mcg of Cytotec at the top of the vagina near the cervix. If 25 mcg of Cytotec did not lead to contractions, neither the cervix nor the baby was ready for delivery. In my experience, 95 percent of my patients would deliver with one 25 mcg dose of Cytotec.

There has been much conflict over the use of Cytotec, because some consider the use of more than 50 mcg of Cytotec a form of induction. The administration of more than 50 mcg of Cytotec has been associated with ruptured uteruses, so some have considered Cytotec too dangerous for induction. In these assessments, there is generally no distinction made between using low doses of Cytotec for cervical ripening or high doses of Cytotec for induction. That's why you need to know how your doctor is using any Cytotec you may be given.

I would like to dispel what I consider to be misinformation about the use of Cytotec. The use of Cytotec for cervical ripening or induction has been criticized because this is an "off label" use of the medication. The "off label" use means the drug is "on label" for some other use in humans and is both safe and effective for use in humans. For example, Depo-Provera was used "off label" for many years. So, it's not as though the "off label" drug in question is unsafe or ineffective in humans. In the case of Cytotec, it is certainly NOT DANGEROUS if DOSED CORRECTLY.

Most all of the Cytotec trials have been on women in hospital labor and delivery rooms. Nurses are instructed to place 50 to 100 mcg of Cytotec into the patient's vagina every two hours. In my practice, I saw my patients in my office, so I could monitor their contractions. I found that the ideal dose was 25 mcg *once*. Labor developed rather miraculously with contractions that were small and lasting for a short amount of time. I would watch my patients in my clinic for several hours to make sure that they were not going into excessive labor, and none of them did. Most of my patients went home for a few hours and then went to the hospital with their cervix dilated 5 cm, as Geena did in the story at the beginning of this chapter.

There is an arbitrary distinction between cervical ripening and induction. I have always used Cytotec strictly for cervical ripening. The purpose of cervical ripening is to get the mother ready for labor. Any use of more than the small 25 mcg dose of Cytotec for cervical ripening becomes an induction. Be sure to discuss the difference between cervical ripening and induction with your doctor.

Today, the balloon method for cervical ripening is increasing in popularity. It's an old method which fell out of style for a while but has come back into fashion. With the balloon method of cervical ripening, a Foley catheter is inserted into the bottom of the uterus and filled with five to ten milliliters of sterile water. This saline-filled catheter is left in place overnight. The balloon is removed the next day. If labor hasn't begun, IV Pitocin is started.

Consider Induction Carefully

There are many good reasons for induction of labor. These include uncontrolled high blood pressure, babies that are large or small for gestational age, women who do not deliver by their 42nd week of pregnancy, fetal death, and abnormal fetal heart rate patterns. But there are conditions in which induction should not be undertaken. These include abnormal presentation, fetal distress, placenta previa, prolapsed cord, women who have had a previous C-section with the classical scar running from the pubic bone up toward the navel, ruptured uterus, and a preterm fetus.

Fifty years ago, Dr. Michel Odent[1] taught that keeping interventions in labor to a minimum allows the baby to decide when he or she is ready to be born, which will start labor. I have always been an advocate of natural labor and allowing the baby to decide when to be born.

Cervical ripening allows your baby to decide when to be born. With cervical ripening, your labor can progress much like a natural labor. If a natural labor is your preferred delivery choice, you will need to talk with your doctor about the difference between cervical ripening and induction.

NOTES
1. Michel Odent, Birth Reborn (Medford, NJ: Birthworks, 1994).

CHAPTER 17

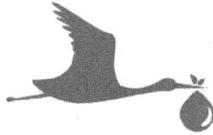

Induction

Intravenous Pitocin is the usual medication used for induction. With induction, you and your physician should start with your cervix being favorable because this will give you a greater chance of being able to have a vaginal delivery. If your cervix is not favorable, your labor will be more difficult, and you may wind up having to have a C-section.

Induction with Pitocin

The most common form of induction is done with IV oxytocin (Pitocin) because it is short acting and therefore can easily and quickly be withdrawn if complications arise. If the Pitocin is stopped because of fetal distress or too many contractions, the problem is relatively quickly resolved because the Pitocin doesn't stay in the blood stream very long. It is important to be able to stop the effect of the induction medications quickly.

Normally, in order to get an effective contraction with Pitocin, you will be given enough Pitocin that you will be unable to stand the pain of the contractions and you will need to have an epidural (injection in your back for pain relief). If this is what you want, you may be satisfied with the induction and the epidural. Some women really don't want to undergo the pain of labor contractions, although without Pitocin, most women can tolerate the pain of normal contractions. In addition, with natural labor, the contractions, besides being less painful, are usually more effective.

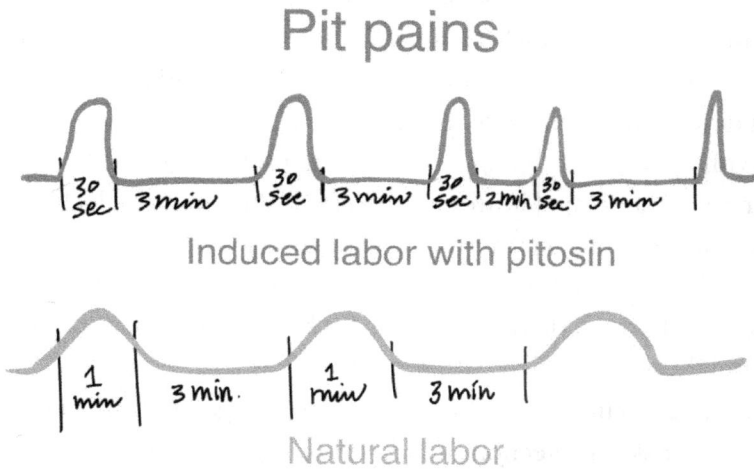

Pit pains

Induced labor with pitosin

Natural labor

Pit pain is the doctor's term for the pain caused by induction with Pitocin. In natural labor, the contractions are more like a bell curve than like a spike. The natural contractions are also more effective than Pitocin-induced contractions and are much less painful.

Speeding Up Induced Labor

Sometimes, induced labor progresses very slowly and your doctor may try to speed up your labor with cervical sweeping or by breaking your amniotic sac.

Cervical Sweeping

If the cervix is favorable but there are no signs of early labor, cervical sweeping can be done. This procedure should be used only for low-risk pregnancies. The mother needs to be at term, the baby's head needs to be in the birth canal, and the mother's cervix needs to be favorable. There should be only one baby. The procedure should not be used with women who have placenta previa or have had uterine surgery, including a C-section with the classical midline incision (up and down rather than side to side).

With cervical sweeping, your doctor inserts a gloved finger into your cervix and runs it around the cervical opening to loosen your amniotic sac from your uterus. In doing this, your doctor helps release prostaglandins, the hormones which helps soften your cervix and prepare your body to deliver your baby. This procedure can be painful and might be associated with some bleeding.

Although many doctors like cervical sweeping, I feel that there is an increased risk for infection of the cervix, especially if the procedure is performed before labor starts.

Manually Breaking the Amniotic Sac

Another technique used to speed up induced labor is the breaking of your baby's amniotic sac. There have been no studies of the long-term effects of manually rupturing your baby's amniotic sac. This sac protects your baby in the same way an egg protects the developing baby bird. If you apply even pressure to the entire eggshell, the eggshell is hard to break. With your baby's amniotic sac, pressure is applied evenly all over your baby's body, providing some protection to your baby's head and neck from your labor contractions.

Consider Your Options Carefully

Your decision whether to have a natural birth or an induction is a complex one. Talk about your options with your physician. During your pregnancy, make a list of pros and cons in your Flight Plan. Your thoughts and feelings about how you deliver may change over the course of your pregnancy. When the time comes for your choice about the kind of delivery you want, you will have considered your options carefully.

CHAPTER 18

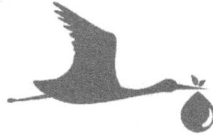

Cesarean Section

For a decade and a half, I worked with thirty family practice doctors when they wanted help with their pregnant patients. I had privileges at four hospitals and did deliveries in all four of them. The end result was that I needed to know not only the styles of the nurses at each individual hospital, but also the style of the physicians making the referrals. I came to recognize that some nurses called frantically for conditions which were not emergencies. Others waited far too long to notify me of emergencies. This particular phone call was of the far too late variety.

"Dr. Lindemann come right away," the nurse said with panic in her voice. "Dr. Lankford has a thirty-five-year-old mother of three in room 108 having fetal distress and the patient is only three centimeters dilated."

"I'll be there in ten to fifteen minutes," I responded.

It was 3 a.m. I got my clothes on as quickly as possible and managed to drive through the blizzard and snowdrifts within fifteen minutes without getting stuck.

I went into Gema's room to check on her. Sure enough, the fetal distress of the baby was visible on the monitor.

There were late decelerations (when the fetal heart rate drops after the contraction).

I now had the task of explaining to Gema and her husband not only what was happening, but also what we needed to do about it. I would have to do an emergency C-section.

"Gema," I said, "your baby is in distress. On the fetal monitor paper, you can see the baby's heartbeat slowing down after your contractions. These decelerations in your baby's heart rate after your contractions indicate *fetal distress.*" I continued, "We need to do a C-section as soon as possible. The anesthetist is getting ready now. I want to do general anesthesia (put you to sleep) because that is the fastest way to get your baby out of harm's way. Your husband can come in with you if you want."

We quickly shielded Gema's eyes from the bright operating room lights, rapidly disinfected her abdomen with betadine, and applied the sterile green drapes. Within five minutes everything was ready.

I gave the order to start anesthesia. One minute later Gema was unconscious. Three more minutes and I had delivered Gema's baby. The baby had good Apgars. I took another fifteen minutes to close Gema's uterus and abdominal wall.

I dictated the operative report, wrote the orders, and then went to see Gema in her room. She was awake. I explained to her that her newborn son had good Apgars and he should grow up to be a healthy man.

Gema was discharged to go home on her third postpartum day in the hospital. She had an unremarkable postpartum course, no depression, no anemia, and no infection.

While I was called in on an emergency basis to deal with Gema's baby's fetal distress, I was able to do an emergency C-section quickly to avoid harm to Gema's baby. Emergency C-sections are sometimes necessary for good outcomes.

When planning for your labor and delivery, a traditional vaginal birth is what most mothers want. Even if you are planning for a vaginal birth, you should become familiar with your other option—the cesarean delivery, or C-section. Sometimes C-sections become necessary on fairly short notice. If you have familiarized yourself with the process and risks of C-sections, you will have a better idea of what's ahead for you in case your plan for a natural delivery gets derailed by some sort of complication.[1]

With a C-section, your baby is delivered surgically. Your obstetrician makes an incision in your abdomen. Most people have no idea how many body layers an obstetrician has to go through to get to your baby. The diagram of the front abdominal wall gives you some idea of the complexity of cutting through many layers of tissue to get to your uterus. There's the epidermis (outside skin layer, which is dead cell tissue), dermis (living skin tissue), subcutaneous tissue, fascia, muscle of the abdomen, rectus muscles (which are separated rather than cut), underneath the separated rectum muscles, more fascia, parietal perineum (sac that holds your stomach contents), visceral peritoneum (covers the uterus), the muscle of the uterus, then the chorion (sac surrounding the amnion), then the amniotic sac—and you're finally to the baby. With all these layers to carefully cut through, it becomes clear why a C-section is major surgery, with the risks associated with major surgery.

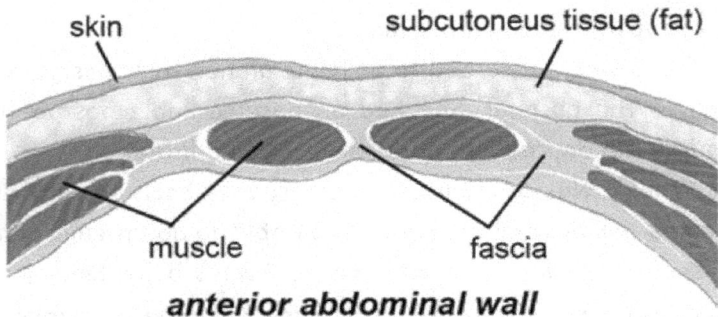

anterior abdominal wall

The important elements of a C-section include timing of no more than twenty to thirty minutes. If the incision is made in the correct place, it can be done with a woman who weighs as little as 130 pounds or one who weighs as much as 500 pounds. The next important part of doing a successful C-section is to minimize cautery (using a heat device to stop small vessel bleeding). Cautery causes necrosis (body tissue dies), which prevents good healing of the incision. The bleeding should stop before the surgery is over if the obstetrician does not cut the arteries in the abdominal wall.

In the United States, over 32 percent of pregnant women deliver via C-section. The risks for a C-section carry all the risks of major surgery, including infection of the inner layers of your abdomen, infection of the incision itself, damage to nearby organs such as cutting a ureter, and post-operative blood clots.

Despite these increased risks with C-section surgery, the C-section has become the most common surgical procedure performed in the United States. You might ask why the C-section rate has increased so much in the past forty years. There are several reasons. A C-section is speedy. It can be done in thirty minutes to an hour. No waiting around for a natural labor to progress through all its stages. More importantly, the obstetrician is paid about twice as much for delivering your baby by C-section than by natural labor. And finally, insurances no longer allow a woman to stay in the hospital long enough for many natural labors to complete. The "failure to progress" diagnosis, followed by various types of induction to speed your labor up, may still not allow you to deliver in the insurance's specified time. By that time, the only other delivery option is a C-section to meet the insurance timeline. This window can be anywhere from twelve to thirty-six hours.

If you want to avoid delivering your baby by C-section (and I recommend you do if at all possible), then you should ask your obstetrician on your initial interview how many C-sections he or she has performed. When I was a resident forty years ago, the normal C-section rate for an obstetrician was 11 percent. Today, a physician's C-section rate should be around 15 percent. If it's greater than this (especially if it hovers around 30 percent), you should consider interviewing other obstetricians if you want to avoid a C-section.

You should also ask what reasons your obstetrician uses to decide a C-section is warranted. Will you be able to deliver twins vaginally? Will you be able to deliver breech babies vaginally? When I was in residency, I was taught how to deliver breech babies and twins vaginally. Today, many obstetricians prefer to deliver breech babies and twins by C-section. In addition, in your early interview with your obstetrician, you should also ask what the C-section rate is for the hospital you will be delivering in. Hospital C-section rates vary remarkably.

Choosing to deliver via C-section can bring a lot of risks, so I still strongly recommend a traditional vaginal birth. I recommend you study your options and discuss them with your obstetrician and make known your preference for a vaginal birth.

NOTES
1. Alan Lindemann, M.D., "How to Do a C-section." Video course. https://lindemannmd.thinkific.com/courses/how-to-do-a-c-section.

CHAPTER 19

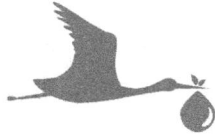

Vaginal Birth After C-section (VBAC)

April had had her first baby by C-section because her baby was breech. She came to the labor and delivery floor in the hospital because her water had broken (spontaneously ruptured membranes).

April asked, "Do you think I can still do a VBAC?"

"Yes, April, I think that is still a reasonable choice for you, but according to ACOG we have some issues to iron out," I explained.

I continued to share with April the things we needed to consider if she was going to deliver by VBAC. "First, the American Academy of Obstetricians and Gynecologists (ACOG) supports the twenty-four-hour rule, that is, delivery is supposed to occur within twenty-four hours after the amniotic sac is broken. With VBACs, the labor and delivery may well go beyond that time period. In addition, ACOG recommends at least one vaginal birth before we try a VBAC."

After reviewing ACOG's recommendations with her, I examined her to determine how ready she was for delivery. "I want to check your cervix at least one time to see whether your cervix is ready for delivery."

I shared my exam results with her. "Good. Your cervix is two centimeters dilated, soft, and thin. I think you are already in early labor. We will do no more cervix checks until we know you are in active labor. You are tall with a large pelvis, and a vaginal birth should be no problem for you."

Twelve hours passed. I checked April's cervix again. "Your cervix is 7 cm, soft, and your baby is head first, not breech."

Two hours later, April delivered a healthy nine-pound baby boy with good Apgars and without an episiotomy.

When I was a medical student forty-five years ago, the management of pregnant women who'd had one or more C-sections was simple: "Once a C-section, always a C-section."

The reason was fear that a uterus would rupture; a medical emergency that most small hospitals cannot manage.

During my third-year medical student obstetrics rotation, a woman who'd had a previous C-section presented to the hospital labor and delivery (L&D) floor. Her cervix was 9 cm dilated, or almost complete. Since she'd had a previous C-section, there was great excitement. The nurses, residents, and staff were in a hurry to send her to the operating room and deliver her by C-section lest she deliver vaginally. This emergency approach made little or no sense to me—even as a third-year student. After all, she and her baby had survived the worst part of her labor. So where was the risk and the emergency?

By the time I returned two years later for my obstetrics residency, some doctors were talking about (and others were doing) vaginal births after C-sections (VBACs). Everyone was cautious, but I had no cause to regret offering and doing VBACs in my residency. There were no maternal mortalities and no emergency C-sections. Not one.

When I arrived at my first practice in 1981, an obstetrician who had immigrated from Canada was a member of the clinical staff. He was pro-VBAC. I read dozens of VBAC articles from other countries—Germany, England, and Scandinavian countries. All reported VBACs to be safe and successful. Despite the often-cited concern about uterine rupture with VBACs, C-sections carry more risk. So, this doctor and I agreed we would offer VBACs to our patients.

The prevailing practice at the time was no induction with VBAC, and we could only offer VBACs to women who'd had at least one vaginal birth before their C-section. A trial of labor (TOL) can be offered women with VBACs, but there is no consensus on what kind of cervical ripening or augmentation should be offered women if the TOL doesn't result in delivery of the baby.

Obstetrics has what is called the "twenty-four-hour rule." Delivery is supposed to occur within twenty-four hours after the membrane (amniotic sac) ruptures. This twenty-four-hour rule is thought to prevent infection in the uterus, cord, and baby. In my experience, it is not the amount of elapsed time, but too many vaginal exams and other manipulations of the cervix, vagina, and baby that cause problems with infection. This includes internal monitors which seem to have come into favor over clinical skills. I was fortunate to have highly skilled clinical nurses when I was doing VBACs.

The fear of induction with a VBAC has been around a long time. ACOG now says induction with Pitocin or a Foley balloon is not a contra-indication for a VBAC. I personally don't like the Foley balloon. In my experience, there seems to be more infection, both maternal and fetal, with its use. I prefer Cytotec (misoprostol) to initiate prodromal labor (the earliest stages of labor).

ACOG doesn't like Cytotec, but in my study of the research—and in my experience—it is not the Cytotec, but the excessive dosing (50 or more mcg) that is the problem. Those studies reporting uterine rupture from Cytotec involved the use of several hundred micrograms of Cytotec over a period of several hours. The routine practice of multiple doses of Cytotec is indeed harmful. Patience and time are the key to success with Cytotec.

As time passed, I became known as the VBAC doctor. Women who couldn't get a VBAC elsewhere sought out my assistance. A nurse midwife who'd had four previous C-sections and no vaginal births came to me wanting a VBAC.

Jackie presented to my office eight weeks pregnant.

"I would like to have a VBAC, but the doctors I work with will not let me even try to have one. I hear you have a lot of VBAC success," she explained.

"Yes, I've done dozens of VBACs for patients. Several of my VBAC patients had had three C-sections," I told her. "No problems have occurred for any of them, not even a blood transfusion." I added, "You know the risks of the VBAC, but you also know the risks of repeat C-sections. I don't see much difference between having had three previous C-sections or four previous C-sections."

Jackie went into spontaneous labor at forty weeks. Delivery was completely unremarkable. She had no epidural and delivered a 7 lb. 1 oz. boy (who was positioned headfirst) without any difficulty. Apgar scores were good and postpartum blood loss was as usual. There was no infection, no blood loss, no episiotomy, and no blood transfusions.

The risk of infection, damaging internal organs, and damage to your baby is greater with a C-section than with a VBAC. From my perspective, VBACs are safe and effective for mothers and babies. I've performed several hundred and supervised others with no maternal or neonatal mortalities—nor any resulting emergency C-sections or hysterectomies.

It's been known for many years that the maternal death rate for planned C-sections is eight times higher than for VBACs. The C-section rate in the U.S. is about 32 percent. We need to bring the

C-section rate down to about 15 percent. VBACs are one way of accomplishing a needed reduction in the C-section rate.

If you are interested in having a VBAC, ask your obstetrician if he or she offers VBAC deliveries. There is an online VBAC organization[1] which could provide you additional information about VBACs and possibly help in locating an obstetrician in your area who does VBACs.

NOTES
1. "Evidence-Based Resource for Birth Options After a Cesarean." https://www.vbac.com/ Online organization providing extensive information about the benefits of VBACs.

SECTION 5

Postpartum Depression

The birth of your child can cause a roller coaster of emotions. It is a happy occasion that makes you feel happy and excited, but on the other hand, you may find yourself experiencing fear and uncertainty. You and your SO might be embarrassed by these feelings, thinking this should be one of the happiest days of your life, but you might not feel that way, so you don't talk about it.

Once pregnant, you are lock-stepped into delivering a baby one way or another.

Delivery is inevitable. This might leave you feeling vulnerable, fearful, angry, frustrated, annoyed, or depressed. Your body is no longer in your control. You may even feel endangered or invaded.

Your ego warns you of danger while your conscious mind says you must like being pregnant, or at least you must not admit that you don't always like being pregnant. Since there is no obvious loss with these feelings, we do not identify these feelings with grief. The issues of this unseen loss are seldom consciously addressed. The popular books on pregnancy simply do not provide much information about the feelings of loss that accompany pregnancy, and how those feelings can result in postpartum depression.

According to the National Institutes of Mental Health, postpartum depression has reached epidemic proportions. An estimated 5 to 40 percent of women giving birth (200,000 to 1,800,000 per year) will develop postpartum depression. The good news is that postpartum depression is treatable. The bad news is the current western medical tradition believes postpartum depression can be neither predicted nor prevented, only treated once identified. Hence, the current western medical tradition believes there are no obvious markers that postpartum depression will develop in patients, and therefore no opportunity to prevent it.

The traditional medical community emphasizes identifying disease and providing drugs to cure the disease. Postpartum depression is no exception. With this gift of new life, your future will bring changes in the order of your day-to-day living which you may find less than welcome. This gift of new life brings with it changes which look in many ways like a trade. Trade implies reciprocation; give and take.

As I often said to my postpartum moms when we discussed this topic, you take the baby and what do you give? You give yourself. Loss involves grieving, and until we look at the grieving component associated with pregnancy and the loss associated with ALL pregnancies, preventing postpartum depression will remain a mystery to the medical community.

CHAPTER 20

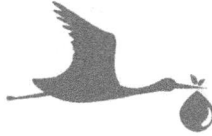

Loss in Pregnancy

One reason postpartum depression is currently not possible to predict is because the many tests for depression look for present depression. If the depression isn't going to develop until next week, the tests will not register any depression. The tests, therefore, have no predictive value. The prevention of postpartum depression will require that we look at the questions we need to ask to allow us to predict and prevent peripartum depression. You want to be able to look for symptoms in yourself and be able to address your depression before it causes problems for you, your baby, and your family.

For over four decades, I have observed what does and does not work for families during and after pregnancy. While I make no claims to psychiatric training, my observations over all these years have allowed me to recognize two areas critical to the strength of your family. All prenatal and postpartum adjustment includes the simultaneous interactions of you and your family on two separate issues:

- changes in your relationship dynamics resulting from pregnancy, and

- your losses associated with pregnancy.

You won't find these two issues on the standard checklist indicating the need to refer a patient to mental health services. Nonetheless, my experience tells me that your conscious attention to these two factors will indicate how well you and your family can adapt to changes brought about by the birth of your baby.

I've talked about the importance of grieving with loss in miscarriage. What isn't talked about is the losses associated with the birth of a baby. Without recognizing the losses and choosing to successfully grieve for them, postpartum depression will remain a mystery.

Elizabeth Kubler-Ross researched grieving associated with loss in the 1960s and described five stages in her book *On Death and Dying*. Kubler-Ross's stages of grief applied originally to death at the end of mature life. She wrote about how normal, successful grieving requires a sequential progression, spending enough time, but not too much time, in each of the stages. Briefly, successful grieving means the sequential progression through all five stages. We have learned a lot from Kubler-Ross. Millions of people have taken comfort by learning to discern their location within these stages. Knowing and anticipating what comes next provides control, security, and therefore comfort. The power from that knowledge validates and affirms you. You begin to know that you are okay. Your knowledge that you are okay supports and promotes your self-esteem.

Based on Dr. Elizabeth Kuebler-Ross's work, there are five now widely-recognized feelings associated with these steps in grieving:

- denial (it's not happening),
- anger (blaming others),
- bargaining (I'll do anything you want if...),
- depression, and
- acceptance (resolution).

The benefits derived from knowledge of the grieving process can be just as appropriately applied to feelings of loss in pregnancy. I believe it is important for you and your healthcare provider to know where you are in these stages of grief, as these same stages are related to the losses associated with pregnancy and postpartum outcomes.

Most people seldom associate birth with loss, but all pregnancies involve some loss, whether you recognize it or not. The grieving cycles associated with both birth and death are remarkably similar. Over the last forty years, I have observed similar grieving cycles in my patients and their families over the kinds of adjustments required with the birth of a baby. Denial, anger, and depression can often arise when your ability to adapt to the changes in your life go awry. When this happens, you are unable to choose to proceed through the steps of grieving. The quality of the choices you make, whether they are made consciously or by default, determine whether or not you will develop risk for depression and ultimately psychosis while you care for your baby.

CHAPTER 21

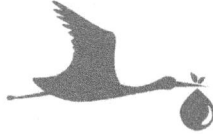

Recognizing Your Loss

Scenario 1:
A Day in the Life of Lisa, Tom, and Baby Alex

5:00 a.m.
Lisa awakened to Tom's alarm. *I'm so tired I don't know how I'm going to make it through this day.* Lisa had been awake for half an hour at 3 a.m. trying to breastfeed baby Alex. *I wonder why he's crying all the time?* Tom's alarm had awakened everybody except Tom. He was very good at pressing the snooze button, so the alarm went off every ten minutes for an hour and a half. Neither Lisa nor Alex could sleep through Tom's alarm, but Tom had no trouble sleeping through it.

6:00 a.m.
Lisa thought, *as long as I'm awake and Alex is awake screaming, I'll try to feed him again.* They sat in the recliner to breastfeed, but Alex had a hard time latching on. He tried to nurse again for ten minutes and then he went to sleep again until Tom's alarm rang again ten minutes later.

7:00 a.m.
For Alex and Lisa, this intermittent breastfeeding and sleeping went on until about 7 a.m. Tom, decided, *I better get up and get ready to go to work.*

7:30 a.m.
Lisa asked Tom, "Could you please set your alarm for 7:00 a.m. since that's when you get up anyway?"

Tom responded, "There you go again complaining about my alarm clock. You know I need to get up to go to work."

When Tom got to the kitchen table, he snarled "You call this breakfast? You know I like fried eggs. Why do you always give me cold cereal?"

"I got three hours of sleep last night. I'm really tired," Lisa said. "Could you take a couple feedings tonight, so I could get more sleep?"

Tom tried to laugh away the request, "Well, you know I can't breast feed."

8:00 a.m.
As Tom was ready to go out the door to work, he angrily asked Lisa, "I'm late for work. Why haven't you ironed any shirts for me?"

Lisa responded, "All I do for my entire day is feed Alex. He doesn't latch on, and my milk isn't coming in. He cries all day long. Then I have meals to make and dishes to do. I just can't seem to get it all done."

"Well Lisa, I've told you before, you're inefficient," Tom replied. "Just put Alex down and let him cry for a while. It's good for him to stretch his lungs. My mom and dad let my little sisters cry and they grew up okay."

Lisa thought to herself *I'm not so sure about that, one of them is in prison and the other one is getting high most of the day.* "Lisa, I have to go to work now," Tom said. "Let's finish this when I get home tonight."

9:00 a.m.
Lisa did the breakfast dishes and Alex woke up screaming again. Lisa thought she would attempt breastfeeding again.

10:00 a.m.
Alex was sleeping. The doorbell rang. It was Lisa's mother, Debbie, stopping in for a surprise visit. She said, "I have nothing to do and I'm so lonesome since your dad died, I thought I would just pop in and hold Alex for a while."

Lisa said, "Mom, I just fed Alex and put him back to bed, but you can help me with the housework. Maybe wash some clothes, clean the bathrooms, or do some ironing."

Lisa's mother said, "I didn't come over here for that."

"I know you didn't Mom," Lisa said. "But I could use some real help."

Despite Lisa's telling her mother that Alex was sleeping, her mother said, "I'm going in to see Alex now. I want to hold him for a while and then I have some shopping to do today."

"Let Alex sleep, please," Lisa said. "Could you pick up some groceries for us so I can rest for awhile?"

"Well, Lisa, I'm not going grocery shopping," Lisa's mother said, "But I tell you what. I'll be back at 2:00 p.m. to hold Alex while you go grocery shopping."

Lisa thought, some help is better than no help. I'll take what I can get.

12:00 p.m.
Alex is awake again and trying to eat. He is still trying to latch on, but he doesn't seem to be very good at it. Lisa has tried a nipple shield, but it doesn't seem to be helping.

They sent her home from the hospital with fifty pages of written instructions and two CDs about postpartum care. She wonders if there is something in there about latching on and babies who cry all the time. Lisa feels like a complete failure, and thinks that perhaps there's a phone number somewhere in all of this stuff for a lactation consultant.

2:00 p.m.

Alex was awake again and screaming. Lisa's mother rang the doorbell. Her mother's reaction was, "You're not going to leave me alone with that are you?"

"Mom, I need a break," Lisa responded. "I'm going grocery shopping. Why don't you manage the best you can? I have a bottle of formula here somewhere."

The nurses in the hospital had told Lisa that she could not give her baby formula if she wanted to breastfeed successfully. For some reason they sent her home with a free can of formula, an appropriate nipple and one bottle, just the same.

Lisa handed her mother the can of formula and the bottle with the nipple and said, "You can try that and see how it works, but I'm going grocery shopping now."

4:00 p.m.

Lisa arrived home with her groceries and carried them into the house. Alex is awake and screaming. Lisa thought, *I'll try breastfeeding again. It's been a while and I'm feeling engorged.* Breastfeeding lasted for about twenty-five min-utes and Alex fell asleep. Lisa placed him in the bassinet in the bedroom. Her mother said, "Maybe you should pick up some formula and do bottle feeding sometimes. That way Tom could help, too."

Lisa had heard of breast pumping, but she didn't have

enough milk the way it was, so she didn't think that would help.

5:30 p.m.
Lisa put chicken, potatoes, and carrots in the oven. She sat down in the recliner and fell asleep.

6:30 p.m.
Tom has come home from work and announced, "I've had a tough day and I'm exhausted."

Lisa replied, "I see you had time to stop by the liquor store and get a 12-pack of beer.

Tom responded, "Well I need something to calm my nerves. Where's dinner. I'm hungry."

"It'll be ready in 10 minutes" Lisa replied.

"Well, I'm going to have a beer and then go play some video games. Call me when dinner's ready," Tom said.

6:45 p.m.
Lisa called to Tom, "Dinner's ready."

Tom yelled back, "I'll be there when I finish this game."

7:00 p.m.
Tom arrived at the dinner table, but the food had cooled down. Lisa had finished eating and Alex was crying again. She picked Alex up and breastfed for another twenty minutes. Alex fell back to sleep and seem to be contented.

7:30 p.m.
Tom was back playing video games again and drinking beer. Lisa returned to the kitchen to do dishes. She asked, "Tom, could you help me do dishes?"

Tom said, "Well I'm busy right now."

8:00 p.m.

Lisa finally had some time to herself, sat down, and fell asleep in the recliner. Tom continued his video games and Alex slept in the bassinet.

9:00 p.m.

Alex was screaming again, wanting to eat. Lisa went to the bassinet, picked him up, and breastfed him in the living room recliner for twenty minutes. Alex went back to sleep in his bassinet on Lisa's side of the bed.

Lisa told Tom, "I'm going to bed now. I want to get some sleep before Alex wants to eat again at midnight. I have been thinking about getting a bottle and some formula so that you can feed Alex, too."

Tom said, "Lisa I'm so busy I don't have time to feed a baby."

Tom played video games until 11:00 p.m. and then went to bed.

12:00 a.m.

Alex was screaming. Lisa got up, took him out of his bassinet, went to the living room recliner, and turned on the light. Alex fed for another twenty-five minutes and went back to sleep. Lisa was so tired at that point that she couldn't sleep and lay awake in bed until 1:30 a.m. when she finally fell asleep again.

3:00 a.m.

Alex was awake again and screaming. Lisa got up, took Alex from the bassinet, went back to the living room recliner, turned on the light, and breast fed for another twenty-five minutes. Lisa's milk was coming in slowly, but Alex had a hard time latching on.

6:00 a.m.
Alex was awake and screaming again. He was hungry. Lisa got up, took him out of the bassinet, and brought him back to the living room recliner. She breastfed again for another twenty-five minutes and Alex went back to sleep. Lisa was about to start another day all over again. She would like things to be different, but she doesn't know what to look for to get what she needs or who to call.

I've said many times in this book, and especially in the depression section, that choosing by default is also a choice: in other words, choosing by default is a choice to not make a choice. I've created two scenarios to show you the difference between consciously dealing with the changes you find when you go home with your new baby and what may happen if you choose to just let things go on as if there's been no changes in your life.

The first story which opens this chapter, "Scenario 1, A Day in the Life of Lisa, Tom, and Baby Alex," is about two parents at home with a new baby. Tom and Lisa have not chosen to consciously create a good working relationship once they arrive home with their new baby, Alex. This story illustrates a couple who do not know they can choose and hence have decided not to decide how to adjust to their new home situation with a new baby.

Most young families are not as dysfunctional as the one in this scenario about Tom, Lisa, and baby Alex. Their story might have been different, more like the second scenario of Jane, Paul, and baby Laurie, if they had taken action to examine critical areas of choice:

- dad attends prenatal visits,

- work out division of labor before the baby is born,

- breastfeeding is important,

- take time out away from home,

- get enough sleep,
- homicide and suicide are occurring during pregnancy and after,
- stop bullying, and
- exit an abusive relationship.

Dad Attends Prenatal Visits

I have always said that 90 percent of getting dad to bond to his wife and child is to welcome him at every single prenatal visit. You and your baby's dad need to understand that there is a little human being in there that is half dad's and that this baby is going to be coming out. Parents need to own their feelings and to own their responsibility before labor and delivery. Bringing mom and dad as well as the other children together for every prenatal visit is an excellent springboard for a safe and happy pregnancy and time at home after delivery. Get ready yo embrace your new life together and embracing your newborn. It goes without saying your life will be changed, but it can be better...not worse.

The person that you were will not return...she or he is lost forever. But you don't have to stay lost. You can work through depression often just by doing the small activities of daily living that I have listed at the end of the first story, Scenario 1. Make your spouse your best friend. Work together with love, respect, and gratitude.

Work Out Division of Labor
Before the Baby is Born

Before your baby is born, you need to talk about division of labor. Who is going to do what, when, and where. Who will feed the baby and when will the baby be fed? Since most newborns are high maintenance, your baby might be hungry every three hours or even more frequently. In the best of all possible worlds, you would know the following:

- how your baby's eating,
- how to get the baby to latch on,
- how much milk you're making,
- when to feed formula,
- when and how to use a breast pump,
- how to store your breastmilk,
- how and when to wash the breast pump,
- who cooks and when,
- who cleans the bathrooms,
- who gets the groceries, and
- how to find and choose daycare.

You need to know all these things before you leave the hospital. If you find yourself at home without answers to the questions about your baby's feeding, you can call your doctor's office or the labor and delivery department at the hospital to find someone who will answer your questions. Another resource could be your mother or father, or your mother-in-law and your father-in-law. They might actually have some good advice, because it's likely they've already been there and already done that.

How is Your Baby Eating?

You should plan on the baby eating five ounces per feeding, maybe a little more or a little less, but when you get the baby home and the baby only wants to eat every four hours, that's great. But that might not happen right away. Often, babies will get only three ounces of milk. And this is from breastfeeding. But the feeding schedule should be fairly well planned out and indelible. If your baby is hungry every three hours, it would be ideal to alternate feedings, at least when dad is on paternity leave or sick or vacation leave. Once dad goes back to work, it is probably reasonable for him to feed the baby at 9:00 at night and 3:00 in the morning.

Although maternity and paternity leave would be welcome, as it is in many civilized countries, in this country we skimp on maternity leave, and we give almost no paternity leave. Dad can, however, often take some vacation or sick leave, which could amount to three or four weeks.

Almost every mom can breastfeed. What sometimes makes breast feeding difficult is anxiety about being unable to breastfeed. You may even breastfeed and pump extra milk. If you do that, dad can bottle feed with breast milk and wash the breast pump.

Some zealous breastfeeding groups recommend no formula, no bottle, and no rubber nipple. Although this works for many women, it doesn't work for everybody. I have found that many crying babies are hungry. If you need to supplement breast milk with formula, don't feel guilty about it.

At six months, your baby should be twice its birth weight. By twelve months, your baby should weigh three times its birth weight. If you have any concerns about inadequate weight gain please consult your pediatrician.

Household Chores

Household chores, preparing meals, cleaning floors, washing clothes, cleaning bathrooms, preparing meals, shopping, and cleaning the breast pump are all considered household chores which need to be divided between moms and dads, preferably before you leave the hospital. You don't want to argue about chores once you get home.

When family members come to visit, let them know that they can help the most by doing household chores or fixing meals. Certainly, they want to hold your baby, but you need to help them understand that you are in charge of the baby, not them.

Time Off

Both moms and dads need time away from home, a night out. Decide when and how long it will be. Everybody deserves some time out.

Get Enough Sleep

If you don't get enough sleep, even making small decisions will seem complicated. Mom and dad will need to decide how to get enough sleep. Work out how you will both take turns sleeping, if necessary, to be sure you are both able to function.

Scenario 2 which follows, "A Day in the Life of Jane, Paul, and Baby Lori," is a story of a young couple who actively chose to succeed with their postpartum life, but they couldn't have chosen had they not known that they could.

Scenario 2: A Day in the Life of Jane, Paul, and Baby Lori

6:00 a.m.

Jane, a twenty-five-year-old first-time mother, heard the cry of her newborn baby girl Lori, but Jane had been awake for ten minutes thinking about the day. *I'm thankful for Paul, my baby Lori, and my eight weeks of maternity leave,* she thought. She looked at her husband, Paul, who had been up at 3 a.m. feeding Lori. Jane had a better understanding than most about what to expect postpartum because she is a nurse working in the obstetric unit in the nearby hospital.

"I'm sure glad I didn't have to get up at 3 a.m. I need sleep to recover from delivery. I'm glad Paul has taken all of his vacation leave for helping with Lori. We can continue with every three-hour feeding. I'll take Lori to the recliner in the living room for breastfeeding while Paul catches up on his sleep," she thought. Jane was looking forward to the time alone with Lori to breastfeed. Paul and Jane planned breakfast at 8:30 each morning, giving Paul time to recover from his 3 a.m. feeding of Lori.

Paul and Jane knew that the American Academy of Pediatrics (AAP) doesn't like the family bed, although that has been the norm for thousands of years. However, the AAP will go so far as to allow a bassinet to be placed beside the parent's bed. Paul and Jane agreed to take turns placing the bassinet beside their sides of the bed so they could monitor Lori during the night. They discovered that sometimes when Lori stirred, just their hand on her tummy would settle her enough to stretch out the time between her feedings to every three hours instead of two.

Jane decided she would breastfeed. Jane knew the routine to try to get a baby to latch on. *I'll put your bottom lip on my areola (the dark of my breast), then place my nipple into your mouth, Lori.* Breastfeeding took twenty minutes. They both fell asleep in the recliner for another half hour.

7:30 a.m.
Jane put Lori in her bassinet, took a shower, got dressed, and prepared breakfast for herself and Paul.

8:30 a.m.

Paul was awake, dressed, and ready for breakfast with Jane. He was thankful for the extra two hours of sleep he got because Jane fed Lori at 6 a.m. Paul said, "Thank you for getting up with Lori this morning so I could sleep in."

Jane said, "Thanks for getting up to feed Lori at 3 a.m. so I could sleep."

They both knew that getting enough sleep is essential for good emotional balance and clear thinking.

9:15 a.m.

Lori was crying again. Jane wanted to weigh her both before and after she ate. Jane knew Lori should be back up to her 7 pounds 10 ounces birth weight by now. She was hoping Lori would get five or six ounces of milk.

10:00 a.m.

Jane's mother decided to drop in for an impromptu visit. "I thought I would stop by and hold Lori for a while," Helen said.

Jane said, "It's always nice to see you, Mom. You're just in time to help with the dishes and vacuum some floors. Lori is just going back to sleep. I'll close the door to her room so that she will sleep more soundly."

Paul said, "Helen, while you are cleaning the kitchen, I'll clean the bathrooms so Jane can get her morning nap. As long as you are out and about, could you run to the grocery store for some eggs, bread, butter, and two chickens?"

Helen said, "Paul, I'd be happy to run to the store. Just let me finish cleaning the kitchen."

11:30 a.m.
Helen returned from the store. "You know, I could just as well make some lunch for the three of us. How about some tuna salad sandwiches and macaroni and cheese?"

12:30 p.m.
Lori woke up, but she wasn't crying. Paul, Jane, and Jane's mother spent the next half hour eating while Lori sat in her car seat on the floor near the dining room table. The next half hour went by without incident. It was Paul's turn to feed Lori. Jane's milk was coming in, but not as much as she needed. Paul heated up formula to room temperature. Lori gobbled down five ounces of formula and went back to sleep. Jane and Paul napped in the living room recliners while Helen cleaned up the kitchen once again. "I'll call you tomorrow to see if you need anything."

Lori's Mom went home. "I'm happy I could help them get through their day so they could get a little rest. I remember how complicated life can be those first few days home with your new baby," she thought.

3:00 p.m.
Lori was awake and whimpering. Jane breastfed Lori without difficulty. After twenty minutes, Lori seemed satisfied and happy. This was a time for mom, dad, and baby to spend some awake time together, cuddling, talking, and reading. Lori remained awake and happy for next hour. Then she went back to sleep.

6:30 p.m.
Lori awakened and wanted to eat again. Jane was happy that her milk was coming in. Lori breastfed again. Lori was awake for another half hour and then went back to sleep.

7:00 p.m.
Time for dinner. This happened to be pizza night. Paul prepared a frozen pizza and served it with coleslaw. Jane and Paul ate and talked.

7:30 p.m.
Jane and Paul spent an hour together sitting on the couch talking, having some quiet time together.

8:30 p.m.
Jane went to bed. Paul cleaned the kitchen and did the dishes.

9:00 p.m.
Lori was awake, but not screaming. Paul fed Lori five ounces of room temperature formula. She was awake for about half an hour. This was a time when Lori and Paul could spend some time relaxing together.

10:00 p.m.
Paul and Lori went to bed.

12:00 a.m.
Lori woke up and wanted to eat. It was Jane's turn. Lori breastfed for about twenty-five minutes. She was awake for another fifteen minutes and then went back to sleep.

3:00 a.m.
Laurie was awake again and hungry. It was Paul's turn to get up with Lori, sit in the recliner, and feed her room temperature formula. Lori ate for twenty-five minutes, then fell asleep again. Paul put her in the bassinet on his side of the bed and they all slept until 6 a.m., when their day begin all over again.

Paul only had five weeks off, so after that, everything would change again. Jane had three months of maternity leave, but she worked at a hospital which had childcare. Jane could then go down to the daycare and breastfeed during the day. Once Jane's milk came in, she could pump so Paul could feed Lori at 9 p.m. and 3 a.m. to help Jane get some rest. Jane and Paul continued to divide the household chores.

The choices we make create who we are. Choice determines our marriage, our wealth, our happiness, our health, our freedom, our strength, and much of our success. As important as choice is, we often make decisions—important ones—without even knowing we are making them. I call that choosing by default. A decision to not decide is still a decision, whether you are prepared for the consequences or not, and those consequences might be less favorable than what you are prepared for or want.

You need to look at the choices you unknowingly make, which can often have surprising and at times negative long-term results. These unrecognized choices can increase risk for depression during your pregnancy and after the birth of your baby.

Grieving is mostly inevitable during pregnancy. Your job is to look at the choices you can make about your grieving during pregnancy so you can intend to have successful grieving instead of grieving without even recognizing it.

The choices you make about grieving during pregnancy and after the birth of your baby can affect how you manage not only your depression after the birth of your baby, but also your long-term happiness, wellness, and relationship success.

CHAPTER 22

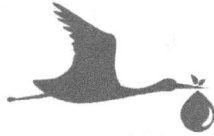

Your Grieving Pattern

The concept that changes in family structure affects relationship dynamics is not new. At weddings, preachers tell us to leave our parents and go to our spouses. This realignment of relationships has been addressed seriously for at least 2,000 years, although I have not seen this change in relationships related to postpartum depression.

Four Versions of Grieving

In my experience, I have observed four versions of postpartum grieving:

- successful grieving with recognized loss,
- successful grieving without recognition of loss,
- unsuccessful grieving with recognized loss, and
- unsuccessful grieving without recognition of loss

While it is important for you to recognize these four varieties of grieving, the most powerful but least noticed is the fourth type, unsuccessful grieving without recognition that loss has occurred, or what I call intangible loss. Intangible loss is less obvious, and you might simply feel that something is wrong. Many families feel intangible loss, but they don't recognize intangible loss for what it is. They don't recognize their feeling as grieving. When we read about suicides and homicides in the paper, we rarely associate these events with the possibility of pregnancy-related intangible loss and unsuccessful grieving.

While tangible loss is obvious, it can still be troublesome unless you, your family, and your doctor choose to guide you to grieve successfully. It's very important that the present support system works for you. I believe it is important for you and your healthcare provider to know where you are in this grieving sequence. In my experience, this sequence is commonly related to postpartum outcomes.

Your Grieving Pattern

While Kubler Ross's five stages of grieving provide you a road map, how you move through these five steps is up to you. Successful grieving depends largely on the way you have been taught to deal with grief by your family. Successful grieving is related to six factors about the way you have been taught to grieve:

1. Your family's grieving model,
2. Desire to grieve successfully,
3. Grief load,
4. Guilt,
5. Shame, and
6. Present support system.

Successful grieving depends upon balance. Envision success like a scale of justice, with side A the successful grieving side and side B the unsuccessful grieving side. If the A side weighs more, you will probably grieve successfully. If the B side weighs more, you may grieve unsuccessfully.

1. Your Family Grieving Model

Your family model is what you learned about grieving from your parents. This is quite likely automatic to you, and while you may not think about it consciously, it's part of your pattern of behavior. When grieving works well, you have no reason to question or even look at how you grieve or whether your model works. When your grieving pattern doesn't work well for you, you need to look at what's going on.

Since your family's grieving patterns are old and automatic, this is the most difficult of the grieving patterns to change.

2. Desire to Grieve Successfully

Choice is the opposite of helplessness. The attitude of helplessness and lack of choice is learned, most likely by example. While you can't always choose your circumstances, you can learn to change your attitude. Decide not to be helpless. Learn to take back your power. Keep your power within your emotional fence where it can be safe and grow.

3. Grief Load

Grieving the loss of your six-year-old child will produce a larger grief load then grieving the loss of your 95-year-old great-grandparent. If you have lost a number of friends or relatives, you may be carrying a heavier grief load than others.

4. Guilt

We usually learn guilt from our families. With guilt, our response is, "I did the wrong thing."

The emotion is associated with something internal. With guilt, anger about the situation you feel guilty about is directed inside of you rather than outside. Anger and depression are similar emotions with a similar amount of energy, but anger is directed outside of you onto something external. This is healthier for you. On the other hand, anger directed internally creates guilt and depression, so it is more destructive to your self-image. Anger directed towards something outside of you protects your self-image. Anger directed against yourself creates depression, which is destructive.

5. Shame

Shame plays a powerful role in grieving because it requires denial on your part, which uses up your energy and decreases your ability to function. Subconsciously you think you have been bad, but you also can't admit it. You pay a high price for defending yourself against these feelings you don't want to have. We put a lot more effort into denial of the shame associated with the feeling "I am wrong or bad" than of guilt because we need to try to bury our shame from our consciousness, protecting ourselves from feeling without value.

Both your guilt and your shame originate in family issues. We all have them. You will be able to grieve more successfully if you understand the correlation between the effectiveness of your grieving and the amount of your guilt or shame you may feel.

Of the four kinds of grieving, intangible loss is the most common kind of grieving associated with the birth of a baby. This kind of grieving is largely associated with a person's inability to adjust to postpartum change. This kind of grieving is also the hardest to diagnose and it's the hardest to treat. Organizations such as Friends of Zane Adams provide extensive information on postpartum depression and hotlines for reaching help.

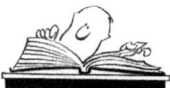

REFERENCES

"Foza Home - Welcome." FRIENDS OF ZAYNE ADAMS - FOZA INC. https://www.fozainc.org/. Extensive resources for finding the help you need for postpartum depression. A nonprofit organization providing supportive resources to families affected by postpartum depression suicides and related maternal mental illnesses.

CHAPTER 23

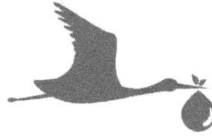

Postpartum Depression is Treatable

During and after pregnancy, anger often arises out of default. If you don't recognize this anger, it can lead to depression by default, even potentially psychotic depression. Denied anger during pregnancy and the depression this denial can bring on will unsettle you, negate you, and weaken you.

Generally, your grieving choices will fall midway between those that are automatic and those you make consciously. As you become more aware of your automatic choices, you can begin to pull into your consciousness some of those decisions you previously made by default. Exercising active choice allows you to greatly improve the quality of the outcomes of your decisions.

Converting Stalled Grieving into Successful Grieving

From my observations of pregnant women and their families for over forty years, I have learned to look at several aspects of what is needed to bridge the gap between what you and your family need and what our social and medical systems are willing and able to provide.

Your Present Support System

Your present support system is not only potentially your best asset, but also your biggest wild card. All the other elements of your grieving pattern fall on either the A or B side of the metaphor of the scale of justice. Your present family support system can reside on either side of the scale, helping or hindering your successful grieving process.

A two-person household relationship is the primary foundation of your family. Communication goes back and forth between two people. Take a close look at how your relationships change before, during, and after pregnancy. With your first child, your family is increasing from two to three people, and it may appear that only one more person is added to your family. However, when a child is added to your family, each parent develops a two-way communication relationship between themselves and the child. There remain the two communication pathways between you and your partner. But there are now four new communication pathways between you and your partner with your child. Overnight, your family communication pathways increase from two to six. The magnitude of this change is unsettling, especially if you are unaware of how these shifts affect your relationships.

Add a second child and you have three other family members with their own communication lines between each other. You are not the only one with additional communication lines. The other members of your family's lines will increase to four each, resulting in twenty-four communication lines between your family members. Sometimes, children will develop a better relationship with one parent than another. You need to recognize, define, list, evaluate, and get ready for these changes in communication.

Risks for Postpartum Depression

There is not one root cause of postpartum depression (PPD). There may be a combination of factors. In my experience, I have found mothers to be at risk for postpartum depression if they experience one or more of the following:

- a history of depression,

- pregnancy or delivery complications,

- history of substance abuse,

- intimate partner conflict, or

- advanced or young maternal age.

Symptoms of Postpartum Depression

This list is not exhaustive list, but these are signs that something is wrong, and you should contact your OB/GYN for an evaluation if you feel this way, even up to a year after you have your baby.

- extreme fatigue,

- low self-esteem,

- sadness, restlessness, anxiety, or hopelessness,

- severe change in appetite,

- mood swings,

- no interest in pleasurable activities

- withdrawal from loved ones,

- thoughts about hurting yourself or your baby, and

- trouble concentrating.

Talk to your doctor about PPD and your risk factors at your first prenatal appointment. It's never too soon to create a safety net of care before and after birth.

Forty years ago, I met a lady who had had seven children and was the wife of a minister. She was late for her appointment.

She apologized for being late. "Sorry I'm late, but I didn't want to take the bus today because people can hear my thoughts. I took my bike."

I asked her, "How long people have been able to hear your thoughts?"

She replied, "Since the birth of my seventh child."

Postpartum depression can last a long time if it isn't recognized and treated. This woman was suffering from a prolonged, benign postpartum psychosis. (The definition of psychosis is a fixed belief which is contrary to reality). By benign, I mean that this patient's prolonged psychosis did not result in the death of her seventh or any of her other children. We commonly think of psychosis as being lethal. The story of the mother who straps her children in their car seats and drives the car into the lake comes to mind. That's a postpartum psychosis which is dangerous for the babies and is an example of unsuccessful grieving and intangible loss (loss of her previous self), as well as tangible loss with the death of her children. The example of the lady who imagined that people could hear her thoughts is a benign postpartum psychosis, but one which continued for twenty-five years. The benign psychosis is most likely the only psychosis that could last that long without resulting in tragedy. Unfortunately, this lady had few mental health resources in her community.

Treatments for Postpartum Depression

Postpartum depression can be treated with psychotherapy, medication, or a mix of both. Psychotherapy will help you and your significant other find better ways to cope with your feelings by talking with a counselor. Your doctor may prescribe antidepressants to help you feel better. If you are breastfeeding, most antidepressants will help you feel better and add little to no risk to your baby. You will have the final decision over your choice of treatment, but consulting with your doctor or a mental health professional will help you choose the best course of action for you.

Pregnancy-related depression can also occur in your husband or significant other. In men, postpartum depression appears later and manifests differently. Depression in men can present as indifference and occurs at about a year after the birth of your baby. Some fathers see the baby as competition for your affection. They can become jealous, indifferent, and seek attention in greener pastures. Fortunately, the medical community is now urging health care providers to check up on any new parent's mental health, regardless of their gender. Your healthcare provider can determine depression or risk for depression if your husband or significant other is present with you for your prenatal visits.

Try Journaling

Years ago, we called "journaling" keeping a diary. Writing down your thoughts and concerns, especially with attention to consciously thinking of things to be grateful for, can help you in many ways. You are more likely to be less depressed, less suicidal, and less anxious. For you, the biggest bonus is improved self-esteem; always a plus, and a very important factor in avoiding depression.

Research indicates that journaling can at times be as good as cognitive behavioral therapy (counseling) for dealing with depression and anxiety. Journaling is a valuable tool to work on lowering your anxiety and depression, especially if you must wait several months for an appointment with a therapist. I recommend starting a journal at the beginning of your pregnancy if you are not already journaling.

Although journaling is very constructive for you, it does not take the place of a counselor. While your journal isn't going to replace your therapist, it's a good way to work through the ups and downs of pregnancy even if you don't need to see a therapist.

You may want to keep two journals, your everyday journal with your private thoughts, and a second journal for issues you want to bring up with your therapist.

In your first or private journal, think gratitude. Gratitude affirms goodness and helps you know that the source of goodness can be outside of yourself. This helps you build a healthy, wholistic view of yourself. In your private journal, each week list three to five causes for gratefulness.

Do not fret about finding new causes for gratefulness. You may use topics more than once. It is personal. You make the calls. Your private journal can often help you find your own answers when you reread your entries. You might also discuss your concerns with your husband or partner. Do not interrupt your flow of thought by trying to control your concerns in your private journal. Vomit them out the first time around. Just get them written.

Your more public journal (your second journal) will help you prioritize the concerns you plan to share with your therapist or your obstetrician. You should prioritize your second journal down to five concerns to present to your doctor. Doctors have been taught to shy away from long lists. Because of present day time constraints, your doctor can't deal with thirteen items. Keeping the list to three to five concerns will allow your doctor to concentrate on your biggest problems.

Choose Successful Grieving

Choice defines us.

You need to look at the choices you unknowingly make which can often have surprising, and at times negative, long-term results. These unrecognized choices can increase risk for depression during your pregnancy and after the birth of your baby.

Grieving is mostly inevitable during pregnancy. Your job is to look at the choices you can make about your grief during pregnancy and how you can choose to have successful grieving instead of grieving without even recognizing it.

Your Flight Plan Beyond Delivery

Most birth plans end with the delivery of your baby. In your flight plan, I encouraged you to consider what you should attend to before you became pregnant, what to attend to during your pregnancy, and of course, what you want in your labor and delivery; the traditional contents of a birth plan.

There is much talk about birth plans and there are hundreds of examples of birth plans online. The thing to remember about birth plans is that they cover a couple of days in your pregnancy. I encourage you to learn what you need to know for a safe pregnancy and delivery, even up to a full year after your baby is born. Some of the worst complications of pregnancy occur after you get home from the hospital. In many other countries, women are followed after the birth of their baby for a full year. I strongly recommend you plan for the consequences of your pregnancy and delivery, not just your day or so in the hospital delivering your baby.

There was a time when new moms were allowed to stay in the hospital until the doctor and the nurses taking care of them felt they were ready to go home. There was time for the nurses to be sure that the new moms were able to nurse successfully. If the doctor and nurses felt the new moms would benefit from another day in the hospital, that choice was available to doctors.

Today, with twenty-four hours the usual hospital stay for vaginal delivery, a bunch of CDs are tossed at the new moms and they are ushered out the door, often before they are ready to deal with the demands of a new baby. For that reason, I strongly advise you to consider extending your flight plan into your days at home with a new baby.

The new baby you are sent home with will change your life forever, whether it's your first or your fifth child. I encourage you to consider how you and your significant other are going to work together to take care of this new life when you get home. Some suggestions include:

1. Before you leave the hospital, have a division of labor plan with your significant other.

2. Crying babies are usually hungry. If your milk hasn't come in yet and your baby is hungry, supplement with formula.

3. Stay regular with prune juice or apple juice.

4. Continue journaling.

5. Watch for the baby blues. If you feel unable to deal with taking care of your baby or overwhelmed, call your doctor. Postpartum depression can develop for up to a year after your baby is born and it can last for decades if untreated.

Air Force One has landed, but don't file that Flight Plan in your memory box just yet!

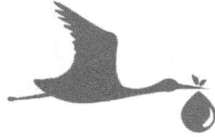

Annotated Resources

A

Acosta, Rina Mae. "Postpartum Care and What We Can Learn From the Dutch." 2015. Finding Dutchland.

https://www.findingdutchland.com/postpartum-care-and-what-we-can-learn-from-the-dutch/

The Scandinavian countries have some of the lowest maternal death rates in the world. This article by an American mother who had her second child in the Netherlands provides much insight on why the Netherlands do birth better than the U.S.

American Association of Birth Centers
https://www.birthcenters.org/default.aspx.

An organization supporting birth centers and midwives in providing an alternative to hospital or home birth. Site appears to be aimed at professionals developing and working for birthing centers, but the organization does have individual memberships and provides a search feature to locate birth centers near you.

American College of Obstetricians and Gynecologists (ACOG)
ACOG. "Preeclampsia and Pregnancy." 2021. https://www.acog.
org/womens-health/infographics/preeclampsia-and-pregnancy
    A very good chart on how to track the symptoms of preeclampsia.

ACOG. "Exercise during Pregnancy." 2022. https://www.acog.org/
womens-health/faqs/exercise-during-pregnancy.
    Presents information on conditions that make exercise during
pregnancy unsafe.

ACOG. Trinidad, Mari Charisse, M.D. and Myra Wick, M.D.
"Neural Tube Defects." *ACOG Practice Bulletin*. Number 187,
December 2017. https://www.maternofetal.net/wpcontent/
uploads/2018/01/Neural-Tube-Defects-MTHFR_ACOG.pdf
    ACOG recommends taking 400 micrograms of folic acid a month
before trying to get pregnant. This bulletin indicates neural tube
closure occurs early in pregnancy. Since at least one half of all pregnancies are unplanned, by the time you know you are pregnant,
you are beyond the stage where neural tubes close. Indicates that
between 16 and 58 percent of neural tube defects could be prevented
by folic acid supplementation. A recent case–control study is cited
that pre-pregnancy folic acid supplementation resulted in a 79 percent
reduction in risk of spina bifida (part of lower spine does not close)
and a 57 percent reduction in risk of anencephaly (part of brain and
skull missing).

American Pregnancy Association (APA). APA. "Birth Centers."
2022. https://americanpregnancy.org/healthy-pregnancy/
labor-and-birth/birth-centers/
    If you are fortunate enough to live near a birthing center, this arti-
cle provides the information you need to compare a birthing center
delivery to a hospital one.

APA. "Exercise during Pregnancy." June 10, 2022.
https://americanpregnancy.org/healthy-pregnancy/is-it-
safe/exercise-during-pregnancy/. Suggestions for guidelines in
choosing various types of exercises while pregnant.

APA. "Headaches in Pregnancy." December 9, 2021.
https://americanpregnancy.org/healthy-pregnancy/preg-
nancy-health-wellness/headaches-and-pregnancy/. Indicates
headaches are common in pregnancy, but most common in first
and third trimesters. Many good checklists to consider in trying to
pinpoint possible causes of headaches in pregnancy.

B

Baby Gaga https://babygaga.com
   Like *First Time Parent Magazine*, there is much information for you
and your family about how to care for you newborn, including pregnancy, baby's first five years, and parenting.

Black Mammas Matter Alliance https://blackmamasmatter.org/
   The maternal death rate for black women is forty-five per 100,000
births—significantly higher than for other ethnic groups. This organization promotes increasing research to reduce the risks of childbirth
for black women.

BPinControl. "Blood Pressure Changes during Pregnancy."
September 1, 2022. https://bpincontrol.in/stress-busters/
blood-pressure-changes-during-pregnancy/
   A site dedicated to all things high blood pressure during pregnancy.
Well worth a visit if you have questions about high blood pressure
in pregnancy.

Boyd, Malinda. "What is Methylation?" 2017. FxMedicine.
https://www.fxmedicine.com.au/blog-post/what-methylation
There is much controversy around MTHFR, testing for it, and treating it. This article is by a naturopath, but it's an extremely clear and easy to understand explanation of the gene variant and how the body's lack of ability to methylate various metabolic processes involving B vitamins. Should be noted that naturopaths often recommend avoiding folic acid, which is a lab-produced form of folate, and instead use a natural form of folic acid called folate.

C

Coalition for Improving Maternity Services (CIMS)
http://www.motherfriendly.org/
A national program to train birth advocates to work with families and hospitals to make birthing more mother-friendly. The CIMS site says their organization is "the nation's largest maternity care consumer advocacy organization." Offers a number of free downloads about their program.

The Commonwealth Fund
https://www.commonwealthfund.org/publications/issue-briefs/2018/dec/womens-health-us-compared-ten-other-countries
Their study indicates that women in the United States have a long history of lacking the health care they need in pregnancy and delivery, with little signs of improvement. In fact, the maternal mortality rate in the U.S. is *increasing*.

ChildrensMD/MomDocs. "Writing a Birth Plan: Ten Essential Tips from a Pediatarician and Mom of 5." 2013.
https://childrensmd.org/uncategorized/

writing-a-birth-plan-10- essential-tips-from-a-pediatrician-and-mom-of-5/

This is an amazingly complete list of things to ask for in your birth plan from a doctor who is the mother of five children.

D

Dailey, Kathleen. "How to Create a Birth Plan." WebMD. 2019. https://www.webmd.com/baby/guide/how-to-create-a-birth-plan

Article assumes this birth plan will be created in the third trimester but contains good information on what to include.

Daniels, Poppy, M.D. "Ten Reasons to Have Your Baby at a Birth Center." 2015. KevinMD. https://www.kevinmd.com/blog/2015/06/10-reasons-to-have-your-baby-at-a-birth- center.html

Gives some of the important ways birthing centers offer a much less interventional approach to labor and delivery than hospitals.

Doheny, Kathleen. "Fixing the Maternal Health Problem in the U.S.: Signs of Hope?" WebMD, December 14, 2021. https://www.webmd.com/women/news/20211214/fixing-maternal-health-problem-us-what-to-know

The maternal death rate in the U.S. is *increasing*. There are many groups studying how to get these numbers down. A very good article about what is happening to improve these numbers, including information and links to the new "Best Hospitals for Maternity" rankings by *U.S. News and World Report*.

E

"Exercise during Pregnancy." Johns Hopkins Medicine. August 8, 2021.

https://www.hopkinsmedicine.org/health/
wellness-and-prevention/exercise-during-pregnancy.
Lists conditions which may make exercise during pregnancy unsafe.

F

"About Factor v Leiden Thrombophilia." Genome.gov.
https://www.genome.gov/Genetic-Disorders/
Factor-V-Leiden-Thrombophilia.
If you have the genetic variation Factor V Leiden, you have a predisposition to develop blood clots in your legs (thrombophelia). Presents a good explanation of the condition and if you have it, much good information about diagnosis and treatment.

First Time Parent Magazine.
http://www.firsttimeparentmagazine.com/
Topics about you, your family, and your newborn after your baby's birth.

"Foza Home - Welcome." FRIENDS OF ZAYNE ADAMS - FOZA INC. https://www.fozainc.org/.
Provides much help with postpartum depression, including hotlines. Highly recommends journaling to help keep a positive outlook.

G

Gere, Helen. "Home Birth vs. Hospital Birth." Family Support America. 2020. http://familysupportamerica.org/
home-birth-vs-hospital-birth/
A lot of good information about the two environments for birthing from a woman who has had a baby in a hospital and is planning on a home birth with her second. Good references as well.

Goldstein, Joelle. "'Beloved' Pediatrics Doctor Dies from Postpartum Complications after Giving Birth to First Child." Peoplemag. PEOPLE, November 5, 2020.
https://people.com/human-interest/indiana-doctor-dies-from-postpartum-complications-after-giving-birth-first-child/

Maternal deaths are largely caused by systems failures because no one person is in charge of your labor and delivery. When physicians die after giving birth for preventable reasons, it becomes very clear what a serious problem the U.S. has in taking care of its women in labor and delivery.

Gunja, Munira Z et al. "What is the Status of Women's Health and Health Care in the U.S. Compared to Ten Other Countries." The Commonwealth Fund. 2018.
https://www.commonwealthfund.org/publications/issue-briefs/2018/dec/womens-health-us-compared-ten-other-countries

The U.S. maternal mortality rate is the highest of all developed countries. This report compares the healthcare provided U.S. women during pregnancy, delivery, and postpartum with the healthcare other countries provide women in these areas.

Gutmann, Amy, M.D. and Jonathan Moreno, M.D. "3 Ways to Empower Yourself to Be Your Best Advocate at Your next Checkup." Thrive Global. August 27, 2019.
https://community.thriveglobal.com/empower-yourself-to-be-your-best-advocate-next-checkup/

Some women find it hard to speak up for what they want in their pregnancies. This article encourages you to do just that.

H

Haelle, Tara. "Why Your Hospital's C-section Rate Can Be Hard to Find." Consumer Reports, 2017.

https://www.consumerreports.org/C-section/
why-your-hospitals-c-section-rate-can-be-hard-to-find/
  You really do need to know if your hospital's C-section rate is higher than nearby hospitals. You may want to choose a different hospital for your delivery.

Harshe, January. Birth Without Fear: The Judgment-Free Guide to Taking Charge of Your Pregnancy, Birth, and Postpartum. Hachette Books, NY, NY, 2019.
  A mother of six children who has experienced C-sections, a VBAC, and home births wants women to know they have options in their pregnancies and shouldn't feel guilty about their choices.

Healthline on Pregnancy
https://www.healthline.com/parenthood/pregnancy
  There is an enormous amount of information here on pregnancy and birth, covering the WebMd kind of topics as well as those more mundane but at times more practical subjects.

Healthline on Birth Plans
https://www.healthline.com/health/pregnancy/birth-plan
  Information on "What is a Birth Plan?" and "How to Create Your Own." This is a very complete list of questions to ask and options to explore for gathering information to include in your birth plan.

Hurley, Judith, RD, MS. "What is a Midwife?" 2020. WebMD.
https://www.webmd.com/baby/what-is-a-midwife

I

Iftikhar, Noreen, M.D. "Headache During Pregnancy: What You Need to Know." 2019. Healthline.

https://www.healthline.com/health/pregnancy/
headache-during-pregnancy
   Information about the kinds of headaches during pregnancy, including what headaches are common during which trimesters, and information on migraines during pregnancy.

Improving Birth
https://improvingbirth.org/
   Providing information on how to make birthing safer for all. Also provides a place where women may anonymously report birthing experiences which went poorly.

Improving Birth Coalition
http://www.motherfriendly.org/
   Information on why we should strive to make birth less interventional.

J

Johnson, Christopher, M.D., "How Safe are Home Births?" A Pediatrician Explains." KevinMD.com, March 30, 2016.
https://www.kevinmd.com/blog/2016/03/how-safe-are-home-births-a-pediatrician-explains.html
   The risk for a home birth is small, Johnson admits. He presents good information on the various ways to look at risk and says that ultimately, the decision to have a home birth depends upon how much risk a woman is willing to take in making the decision for a home birth.

L

LactMed. "Drugs and Lactation Database (LactMed)." National Library of Medicine.
https://www.ncbi.nlm.nih.gov/books/NBK501922/

The LactMed® database contains information on drugs and other chemicals to which breastfeeding mothers may be exposed. It includes information on the levels of such substances in breast milk and infant blood, and the possible adverse effects in the nursing infant. Suggested therapeutic alternatives to those drugs are provided, where appropriate. All data are derived from the scientific literature and fully referenced. A peer review panel reviews the data to assure that the information is accurate.

Lamaze Organization
Home: https://www.lamaze.org

"Fitness During Pregnancy."
https://www.lamaze.org/pregnancy-fitness.
The Lamaze organization is known primarily for its support of breastfeeding women. However, their web site has much valuable information about many topics helpful for pregnant and nursing women. This particular article provides a helpful discussion of the advantages of fitness in pregnancy and types of exercise by trimester.

Library of Congress. Home. https://www.loc.gov
The Library of Congress is an amazing collection of print resources, from transcripts of congressional hearings to housing a copy of every book published in the United States. The holdings occupy three buildings, and the site provides a video tour of all three. With a source this vast, it may take a while to find information on what you are researching, but there is a search bar. A search on books and printed material on maternal mortality returned 1,294 items, with 874 available online.

Lindberg, Sara. "Safe Pregnancy Workouts: Best Exercises by Trimester." Healthline. Healthline Media, April 30, 2020.

https://www.healthline.com/health/pregnancy/
pregnancy-workouts.
Makes suggestions for best exercises by trimester.

Lindemann, M.D., Alan. "Interview with Family of the Quads Delivered by Dr. Lindemann." 2020. YouTube.
https://www.youtube.com/watch?v=iTcdOGVnTfk&t=29s
This is a YouTube video. It is almost an hour long, but Dr. Lindemann has made a transcript of the video available on Scribd at https://www.scribd.com/document/472658166/quads-copy-docx

M

Major, Mandy. "What Postpartum Care Looks Like Worldwide, and How the U.S. Compares." 2020. Healthline.
https://www.healthline.com/health/pregnancy/
what-post-childbirth-care-looks-like-around-the-world-and-why-
the-u-s-is-missing-the-mark#Rights

March of Dimes (MofD)
Home: https://www.marchofdimes.org/
https://www.marchofdimes.org/pregnancy/pregnancy.aspx
This organization has been around for a long time and many people still associate it with development of a vaccine for polio. However, the organization has taken on researching many areas of pregnancy and birth and now considers its mission to be fighting for the health of all mothers and babies.

MofD
Good discussion of birth plans.
https://www.marchofdimes.org/pregnancy/your-birth-plan.aspx

Also offers an excellent three-page plan ready to be filled out. https://www.marchofdimes.org/materials/March-of-Dimes-Birth-Plan 2020.pdf

MofD. "Nowhere to Go: Maternity Care Deserts Across the U.S. 2022."https://www.marchofdimes.org/maternity-care-deserts-report
    A report on counties in the U.S. which lack maternity care and how to cope with living in an area lacking maternity care.

MofD. "Folic Acid." May, 2020. https://www.marchofdimes.org/pregnancy/folic-acid.aspx#.
    While most folic acid recommendations are for 400 mcg folic acid a day before pregnancy, if you know you have MTFHR, you should take 4,000 mcg of folic acid before and during early pregnancy. It can help reduce your risk of having another baby with a neuro tube defect by about 70 percent.

Maressa Brown, C. W. E. (2022, December 15). *Delivering at a birth center. What to Expect.* https://www.whattoexpect.com/pregnancy/birth-center/
    Very thorough assessment of experiences at birthing centers as opposed to hospitals.

McClurg, Leslie. "Home birth can be appealing, but how safe is it?" 2019. National Public Radio. https://www.npr.org/sections/health-shots/2019/03/11/700829719/home-birth-can-be-appealing-but-how-safe-is-it
    Another good discussion of the pros and cons of home birth, with a comparison of the costs.

Medline Plus. "MTHFR Mutation Test." https://medlineplus.gov/lab-tests/mthfr-mutation-test/

Another good explanation of what the MTHFR mutation is and the kinds of problems it can cause.

Murkoff, Heidi. 5th ed. *What to Expect When You're Expecting.* Workman Publishing, New York, 2016.

This is the Dr. Spock (not the one with pointy ears), the pediatrician who many years ago wrote an encyclopedia of topics to let parents know how to raise their children. Heidi Murkoff has written the Dr. Spock of pregnancy. Here's where to read about whether you should eat sushi or not while you're pregnant.

N

National Academies of Sciences, Engineering, and Medicine. *Birth Settings in America: Outcomes, Quality, Access, and Choice.* Washington, DC: The National Academies Press, 2020, 368 pages. https://nap.nationalacademies.org/catalog/25636/birth-settings-in-america-outcomes-quality-access-and-choice

The Academy books are available in hard copy for a price. Don't be put off by the price listed for a hard copy. You may download a pdf copy of the book for free. There are 354 pages here, with an abundance of information on who served on the committees. Scroll on down to the table of contents where you will find the meat of the book. When you are trying to decide where you want to delivery your baby, this book supplies research information on how the birth setting influences your labor and delivery.

National Headache Foundation. https://headaches.org/

Not confined solely to headaches in pregnancy but offers a very large list of headache tools, and much information on migraines. Also provides a list of clinical trials.

National Institute of Office of Dietary Supplements. "Folate: Fact Sheet for Consumers."
https://ods.od.nih.gov/factsheets/Folate-Consumer/
  Good discussion of how our body uses folate, what foods we find folate in, and the various forms of folate used for supplementation.

O

Odent, Michel. *Birth Reborn*. Souvenir, 1994. An old book, but Odent played a prominent role in developing the notion that a baby should be able to decide when to be born.

Oster, Emily. *Expecting Better*. New York: Penguin Books, 2018. Explores some of the conflicting research on pregnancy, presents the results of the studies, and encourages you to decide what you think is best for you.

P

Planned Parenthood. "What is Ectopic Pegnancy?: Definition and Treatment."
https://www.plannedparenthood.org/learn/pregnancy/ectopic-pregnancy
  The Planned Parenthood website has information about the risk for women to develop an ectopic pregnancy.

Pregnancy by Design
Organized by professionals in childbirth and maternal health to provide expecting parents with quality information about pregnancy and birth.

"Why Do Birth Plans Fail?"
https://pregnancybydesign.com/why-do-birth-plans-fail/
Many women who have traumatic births had a birth plan, but for some reason, the birth plan didn't result in the kind of birth envisioned. This article focuses on ways birth plans to fail and how to avoid problems if at all possible.

R

Red Tricycle
https://redtri.com/national-kids/
Billed as things to do with kids, this site has a lot of information on pregnancy as well.

Runners World. "Everything You Need to Know About Running While Pregnant." 2023.
https://www.runnersworld.com/training/a20849722/
what-you-need-to-know-about-running-and-pregnancy/
Guidance from runners about running while pregnant.

S

Stegenga, Jacob. "Gentle medicine could radically transform medical practice." *Aeon*, 13 May 2020.
https://aeon.co/ideas/how-gentle-medicine-could-radically-transform-medical-practice
John Stegenga discusses several of the practices in medicine today which have created a highly invasive medical culture. Unfortunately, obstetrics has become one of those medical specialties with growing interventions, especially C-sections.

T

ThirtySeconds.
https://30seconds.com/pregnancy/
    Website with information on all aspects of pregnancy, including articles on fetal development. Much information on many issues surrounding pregnancy.

U

USA Today Investigations. "Advocate for Yourself: Lifesaving Tips for A Safer Birth."
https://www.gannett-cdn.com/experiments/usatoday/responsive/2018/maternal-harm/graphics/life-saving-tips.pdf
    It's not often that unsigned, undated information can be relied upon, let alone helpful. However, this two-page list of tips for keeping you alive during your birth is excellent, including information on checking that your blood loss is measured after delivery. Sources for the information are listed as: Sources : AIM Program, CMQCC, ACOG, Preeclampsia Foundation, and USA TODAY research.

V

VBAC—A Safe Alternative to Repeat Cesarean.
https://www.vbac.com/
An enormous amount of information in support of VBACs as a safe alternative to a repeat C-section.

W

WebMed.
Home: https://www.webmd.com/

WebMed. "How to Create a Birth Plan." 2019
https://www.webmd.com/baby/guide/how-to-create-a-birth-plan#1

There are many sources for information on birth plans, but WebMed provides a good summary of what should be in a one.

WebMD. "What is a Midwife?" 2023.
https://www.webmd.com/baby/what-is-a-midwife#:~:text=A%20midwife%20is%20a%20trained,no%20complications%20during%20their%20pregnancy.

Very good discussion of midwives and other birthing roles for support in pregnancy, labor, and delivery.

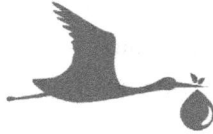

Acronyms

AAP	American Academy of Pediatrics
ACOG	American College of Obstetricians and Gynecologists
ALT	alanine amniotransferase
ALP	alkaline phosphatase
AST	aspartate aminotransferase
BMN	serum neutrophils
BP	blood pressure
BUN	blood urea nitrogen
CAT	computer aided tomography
CDC	Center for Disease Control and Prevention
CEO	Chief Executive Officer
CD	compact disc
D&C	dilation and curettage
D-dimer	test for protein fragments from blood clots
DNA	deoxyribonucleic acid
DVT	deep vein thrombosis
ECV	external cephalic version
EL	elevated liver enzymes
ER	emergency room
FVL	factor 5 Leiden
HCT	hematocrit

HELLP	hemolysis, elevated liver enzymes, and low platelets
IUD	intrauterine device
IV	intravenous
Hgb	hemoglobin
hyperalimentation	fluids by IV or NG-tube
leukocytes	white blood cells
L&D	labor and delivery
LFTs	liver function tests
LP	low platelets (white blood count)
MTHFR	methylenetetrahydrofolate reductase
NG-tube	naso-gastric tube (inserted through nose)
NST	non-stress test
NTD	neural tube defect
OCT	oxytocin challenge test
platelets	white blood cells
Rh	rhesus factor
SO	significant other
STD	sexually transmitted disease
TOL	trial of labor
VBAC	vaginal birth after C-section
WBC	white blood count

Acknowledgments

Like most writers, we have been working on this book for over three years and often wondered if we would ever get it done. Writing and publishing a book is much different than it was thirty years ago when we wrote *Modern Medicine: What You're Dying to Know.*[1]

Can you really tell when a book is born? We believe this book was born when we were fortunate enough to be able to interview Sandy and Doug Powell and their four children, quadruplets, which I delivered in January of 1997. Sandy had been kind enough to send me Christmas cards every year with pictures of the quads. I wanted to interview Sandy and Doug about what it was like to raise quadruplets, and Sandy said the quads wanted to be included. What a gift! We talked for an hour and that got me thinking it was time for me to write a book about safe pregnancy.[2]

From the beginning, I was fortunate to be able to connect with Steve Harrison and his team which supports writers, including Jack Canfield. They read what parts of the book we had completed and were always there to let us know what worked and what didn't. Other members of Steve's team jumped in to help. Geoffrey Berwind on storytelling. Deb Englander on developmental editing. Cristina Smith on author coaching. Valerie Costa on copy editing. Christy Day for book layout and design.

Even with Steve's incredibly rich resources for writers, I still didn't have an understanding of all the steps necessary today in publishing a book. Another Harrison team member, Sarah Brown, stepped up to the plate and picked up the pieces of my manuscript and walked me through the step-by-step process of publishing today. This book wouldn't be in your hands had I not had the help of Sarah Brown and Steve Harrison's team.

NOTES
1. Lindemann, Alan R. and Diane Haugen. *Modern Medicine: What You're Dying to Know: A Consumer Action Guide*. Elgin, ND: ARL, Inc., Reprint 2020.

2. Interview with the Powell family on YouTube.
https://www.youtube.com/watch?v=iTcdOGVnTfk

About the Author

One of the things I learned as a medical student and resident is that in obstetrics you can have a lot to say about your outcome. In other words, you can pick your outcome much of the time—not all of the time—but certainly about 90 percent of the time. Pregnant women so often feel they shouldn't question the expert, the obstetrician. My goal is to provide pregnant women a safe arena where they can freely ask questions about their choices in their pregnancy and delivery. I can't offer you medical advice, but I can share with you my experiences with the 6000 babies I delivered.

In today's medical environment, it is very difficult to raise questions about your choices in your health care. I want to encourage women to have the confidence to trust in themselves and the decisions they make about their care.

My patients helped me gain valuable insight into what turns a high-risk pregnancy into a low-risk one, and how to keep a low-risk pregnancy low risk. You won't find this information in medical texts. I have learned a lot over my years of delivering babies and I want to share this information with you. Your safety as a patient may well depend upon your knowing the things I talk about in this book.

My goal is for every pregnant woman to have access to the kinds of information needed to guide her pregnancy and delivery towards the best possible outcome for herself and her family.

www.ingramcontent.com/pod-product-compliance
Lightning Source LLC
Chambersburg PA
CBHW060040030426
42334CB00019B/2407